POWER EATING PROGRAM
You Are How You Eat

POWER EATING PROGRAM

You Are How You Eat

Lino Stanchich

Healthy Products, Inc.

Original edition © 1989 by Lino Stanchich
Healthy Products, Inc.
P.O. Box 19315
Asheville, North Carolina 28815
(828) 299-8657

All rights reserved. Printed in the United States of America.
No part of this book may be reproduced in any form or by any means
without written permission from the publisher.

Note To The Reader: Those with health problems are advised to seek
the guidance of a qualified medical or psychological professional in
addition to a qualified macrobiotic teacher before implementing any
of the dietary or other approaches presented in this book. Neither this
nor any other related book should be used as a substitute for qualified
treatment.

First edition: October 1989

Library of Congress Catalog Card Number: 89 - 085504
ISBN 0 - 9624114 - 0 - X

Illustrations by Jane McElroy

Quote from Dr. Robert Haas reprinted with permission of Rawson Associates,
an imprint of Macmillan Publishing Company from *Eat To Win, The Sports
Nutrition Bible* by Dr. Robert Haas. Copyright © 1984 Robert Haas.
Quotes from *Code of Jewish Law* reprinted by permission of the publisher,
Hebrew Publishing Company, copyright © 1963. All rights reserved.
Quotes from *Take A Deep Breath* by James E. Loehr, Ph.D. and Jeffery A.
Migdow, M.D. reprinted by permission of Jerome Agel, 2 Peter Cooper Road,
New York, New York 10010. Copyright © 1986 by Jerome Agel.
Quote from Swami Muktananda, *Satsang With Baba*, Vol. I, 85-87. Copyright
© 1974 SYDA Foundation. All rights reserved. Reprinted by permission.
Quote from Swami Muktananda, *Reflections Of The Self*, Part I, v. 198.
Copyright © 1980 SYDA Foundation. All rights reserved. Reprinted by permis-
sion.

10   9   8   7   6   5

This book is dedicated to my parents,
Antonio and Giovanna Stanchich,
who gave me life and a foundation
of strength and love.

ACKNOWLEDGEMENTS

I would like to thank:

My teachers George and Lima Ohsawa, Michio and Aveline Kushi, Noboru Muramoto, Herman and Cornelia Aihara, and Shizuko Yamamoto for your inspiration, knowledge, guidance, and friendship.

Robin Brown and her husband Bill Younkin for your generosity, patience, expertise, and encouragement.

Stephen Fuller-Rowell, who offered the original motivation for writing this book.

Jackie and Sandy Pukel and all my students and friends at the Macrobiotic Foundation of Florida and Macrobiotic Centers of Florida, for your friendship and support.

Nancy Quinn Moore for your expert editing and most of all for your positive attitude and encouragement.

Marquita and Warren Wepman with whom we enjoyed many meditative meals, for your special friendship.

Alix Landman for your expert advice on nutritional information and for your friendship.

Phyllis Slotkin, one of my best assistants and most devoted students, for your dedication and valuable suggestions for this book.

Jane McElroy for the gentle energy of your lovely illustrations.

Marilyn Burrows for your spirit, enthusiasm, and advice.

Sunny Emerson for your careful proofreading and persistence in encouraging me to write this book.

Jane Quincannon without whom this book would never have materialized, for your hard work, insights, and devotion.

All my students worldwide who have given me the priviledge of sharing your experiences, courage, wisdom, and friendship.

For all of you I feel deeply blessed.

CONTENTS

FOREWORD

Lino Stanchich is a wonderful person who, for two decades, has been continuously dedicated to the development of humanity and the betterment of our social, physical, mental, and spiritual well-being. Lino offers this book, *Power Eating Program* to everyone. Every reader will benefit from Lino's contribution to our health, freedom, and happiness.

Michio Kushi
Brookline, Massachusetts

I was first introduced to the importance of eating and chewing in 1950 when I visited George Ohsawa's dormitory near Tokyo. Ohsawa was teaching that whole natural foods, like those eaten by traditional cultures in the past, were the basis of personal health and peace in society.

When I came to America several years later to teach macrobiotics, we started to teach the importance of these foods. The natural foods movement is now well underway in this country and in Europe. I recently have become interested in other important aspects of healthy eating—the amount of food we eat and the way we eat.

I am happy that Lino Stanchich has written this basic guidebook on how to chew. Lino has made valuable information available on a subject of prime importance in macrobiotic practice.

Chewing helps us to be modest and to appreciate the foods we are given. Without chewing well, information about diet and health is of little value. Chewing is so simple that it is easy to forget.

I thank Lino for reminding all of us just how important it is. As you will discover, the key to health and happiness is in our hands. I hope you will enjoy this book and begin chewing well, starting with your next meal.

Aveline Kushi
Brookline, Massachusetts

Place yourself in the middle of the stream of power and wisdom which flows into you as life, place yourself in the full center of that flood, then you are without effort impelled to truth, to right, and a perfect contentment.

Ralph Waldo Emerson

For God hath not given us the spirit of fear; but of power, and of love, and of a sound mind.

Paul the Apostle to Timothy 1:7

PREFACE

Power, the first word in my book, represents our inner life force, the energy which flows through all things. When used with consciousness and love, power creates health, happiness, and peace. The way you eat affects you physically, mentally, emotionally, sexually, and spiritually. The Power Eating Program will teach you how to experience and develop your greatest potential of power each time you eat.

In a German concentration camp during World War II, my father made a miraculous discovery that enabled him to survive. After his liberation, he taught me this amazing discovery. Ironically, it later saved my life. My father's simple yet profound lesson is the foundation of this book.

The goal of the Power Eating Program (PEP) is to help you become a healthier, happier person who not only survives but thrives! The solutions to life's problems are rarely mysterious or hidden. The key to health is right under our noses, three times a day. Stop and reflect upon your eating habits. Consider the changes you want to make in your life.

When properly practiced, PEP will help maximize your as-

1

similation of food and improve your digestion. The Power Eating Program will help you eat less and eat fewer times a day. It will boost your body's immune system, increase your vitality, and it may save you money. It might even save your life.

The Power Eating Program is a step-by-step guide to achieving optimum value, not only from your meal, but your mealtime. *How* you eat is as important as *what* you eat. You will learn why you eat, when to eat, how to transform food into energy, and what foods supply the most healing power. To put the Power Eating Program in perspective, I have included abundant data, quotes, and opinions from renowned experts in the health and personal transformation fields.

For the past twenty years, I have counseled thousands of people who have tried many health programs and diets with poor success. Yet, after having learned *what* to eat and *how* to eat properly, they began to improve and to heal themselves, often of "terminal" illnesses. Experience has shown that when healthy people practice PEP, they frequently feel the benefits after one meal. Those who eat a macrobiotic, vegetarian, or Pritikin-type diet will experience the most positive health results.

If we are to nuture our bodies and our planet, we must change. The time has come for adopting a way of eating that is ecological, healthful, non-violent, and balanced. The only way to absorb such a diet is to eat it properly. Few of us learned this as children.

Health and transformation require discipline and awareness. This book will provide you the information and, I hope, the inspiration to make the changes you want in your life. Eating well is a powerful way to love ourselves.

Lino Stanchich
Miami, Florida, September 1989

INTRODUCTION

In 1943, during World War II, my father Antonio Stanchich was taken prisoner in Greece by the Germans and sent to a concentration camp in Germany. The camp was connected to a factory where all the prisoners were forced to work very hard.

The weather in winter was cold. The barracks were poorly heated, clothing was inadequate, and the food was substandard. My father told me, "I was cold most of the time and hungry all of the time."

In the morning my father received one cup of chicory coffee and one slice of bread. For lunch and dinner he was given one bowl of soup. The soup was made of potatoes and some other vegetable and included grain or bean, and occasionally a bit of meat. People died of starvation daily. During the cold winter months, death due to exposure increased considerably. Life in the camp was a constant fight for survival.

Then my father made a discovery that would save his life. When he was thirsty, he intuitively retained the cold water in his mouth and chewed it a while to make it warm before swallowing it. He usually chewed his water 10 to 15 times. One day when the water was very cold, he chewed it 50 times!

Aside from quenching his thirst, the water actually seemed to give him energy. At first he felt it was his imagination but after several experiments he concluded that, indeed, chewing water 50 times or more gave him more energy. He was puzzled. How could plain water give him energy? Forty years later, this mystery was clarified.

My father began an experiment. In the beginning, he chewed his food only 50 times a mouthful, then he tried 75, then 100, 150, 200, even up to 300 times a mouthful ... sometimes more. He told me that the magic number of chews was 150 times and after that he could chew almost indefinitely with steady increases in energy. Often there was little time to chew. The morning meal lasted one half-hour. Lunch was one hour long, but dinnertime lasted as long as he wanted.

The technique my father developed was simple: Place one tablespoon of liquid or solid in the mouth and chew, counting each chew. He shared his discovery with his friends, most of whom told him, "Come on, Tony, that's all in your head!" His friends thought that 10 to 20 chews were enough, yet two of them joined my father in his chewing sessions and they compared notes. They all concluded that this technique gave them more energy. They felt less hungry and even more warm.

After two years in the concentration camp, the prisoners were liberated in 1945 by the American Army. A few months later, my father came home to us in Fiume-Rijeka, formerly Italy, now Yugoslavia. He was skinny but alive. Of his ship's crew of thirty-two who were captured and sent to the concentration camp, only three survived. *Those who lived were my father and his two friends who practiced chewing.*

The following year, while on a family picnic, my father shared with me his experience at the concentration camp. He attributed his survival totally to chewing. He closed his story by telling me, "If ever you are weak, cold, or sick, chew each mouthful 150 times or more." I was 14 years old at the time. There was plenty of food in our house in 1946 and I was in good health. However, I never forgot his words.

In 1949, Yugoslavia was in political turmoil. Its communist government did not allow Italian citizens to travel to Italy. Many who opposed the government tried to escape from Yugoslavia. That year, on the 10th of March, I attempted to escape and was captured at the border and sentenced to two years of hard labor.

At seventeen, I too was a prisoner.

While not as horrible as the German concentration camp in which my father was imprisoned, my time in prison was extremely difficult. The diet was similar to my father's: one bread roll with chicory coffee for breakfast; one bowl of soup, usually with barley and beans for lunch; and the same for dinner. Once a week the soup had some meat in it. I considered the meal good if there were 20 beans in the soup. I, too, was hungry most of the time.

A crucial difference between my father's experience and my own was that I was allowed one small package a month from home. Because parcels often did not arrive, I requested that my mother send me raw onions, salt, and dried, sliced whole wheat bread. I felt that no one would steal such a package and sure enough I received them all.

This supplementation made all the difference. I would slice the onion in wedges, dunk the wedge in salt, and chew it with a piece of dried bread. Followed by one to two glasses of water, this would fill me up. When properly chewed, it gave me great energy and a strange feeling of confidence and courage. I simply was not afraid of anything or anyone.

I chewed the way my father taught me, up to 150 times or more, with one important addition. I chewed with my eyes closed. The results were excellent. I successfully avoided taking in the depressing surroundings. In addition, closing my eyes internalized my energy. By not looking outward, my energy went inward, strengthening me even more.

My experience in the concentration camp affected me deeply. I changed from a lighthearted, jovial young boy into a hardened, tough man. When I arrived home in 1951, looking much older than my nineteen years, my brother remarked, "If I didn't know you and saw you in a dark street, I would give you my wallet without your asking for it."

One year later my family was allowed to go to Italy and in 1953 we emigrated to the United States. Food was plentiful in America. Along with my brother, I owned and operated several restaurants. With the rich American diet, there was no thought of starvation. I stopped my chewing regime.

Many years passed and I went through a number of changes until 1969, when I began to suffer the detrimental effects of my high-stress life. I came to the startling realization that *I was digging my own grave with my fork!* Nutrition and health foods became an interest of mine. I tried many diets, from raw foods to fruit only, from high protein to lacto vegetarian. All worked temporarily. Then I discovered macrobiotics, which I enthusiastically studied and adopted. I was once again determined to survive.

Through what we consume, we change the quality of our body, mind, and spirit. Each of us is responsible for his or her own life and destiny. We are our own masters, and no one else can chew for us.

Michio Kushi
The Book of Macrobiotics

...The body is the product of the food that you eat. And the inner psychic instrument—the mind, imagination, intellect, and ego—are also products of the food you eat....Food is life....Food is realization. And food is heaven as well as hell.

Swami Muktananda
Satsang With Baba

POWER EATING PROGRAM
YOU ARE *HOW* YOU EAT

Food seems to be the "Final Frontier." When people experience imbalances in their health, they try counseling, divorce, relocation, pills, herbs, and surgery. Then as the last resort, they try to change their eating habits as an "after-all-else-fails" attempt to regain their health. When we eat food in a conscious manner, we may, as Hippocrates, the Father of Medicine taught, "Let food be thy medicine, and medicine be thy food."

Eating is a primal desire, the basis of our survival instinct. So simple an act, eating is underestimated as a major influence on health. Yes, there are other vital influences, yet if you question the importance of food, try fasting for several days, or notice the response of a hungry infant. As with all basic human functions, eating can be a greedy indulgence or a spiritual experience. Our choice of how we eat can merely fill us up and comfort us, or it can heal and transform us.

7

In many traditions and cultures, eating is considered an extremely important, even sacred act. I was told by a friend from Lebanon that an ordinary peasant is not required to stop eating even if a king enters his house. Also, ancient Jewish Law states that if a piece of food larger than the size of an egg is eaten, one must sit down and say grace. Eating with a reverent attitude is recommended in many spiritual practices.

Yet these days we casually interrupt our meals for the telephone, other people, and all the thousands of hectic, chaotic influences of modern life. While we eat, we're jumping up and down, talking, reading, "grabbing a bite" and then grabbing a digestive tablet. According to *Consumer Spending Report*, Americans now spend over *$1 billion* on digestive medicine each year! Some people are suffering. Take a good look at *your* life-style.

Michael Rossoff, an expert acupuncturist, macrobiotic counselor, and teacher, writes in a *Solstice* article entitled, "Finding Peace of Mind in Troubled Times":

> The experience of eating, where the aromas, colors, textures and tastes combine to fill our senses and stomach, is for many a forgotten skill. If you are watching television, reading a magazine or driving a car while eating, you inevitably miss the wholeness of a meal. No wonder so many people either overeat or are chronically hungry.

We scurry like rats in a maze, at great detriment to our health. If foods are the building blocks of our health, then the stressful U.S. mealtime habits are causing our country to crumble. Americans are overfed and undernourished. For too many people, food has become a form of entertainment rather than a means of nourishment. Smiling clowns sell brightly colored boxes of high-fat, sugary foods. Cartoon characters, film stars and athletes convince Americans to eat junk food.

Yet a growing number of Americans are changing their eating habits. Unfortunately, some people who eat a healthy diet achieve insufficient results, and they cannot understand why. In most cases, the reason is that they are concerned only with *what* to eat and forget about or have never learned *how* to eat. Very few people I observe know how to obtain the full power from their food. The effects of even the most healthy meal can be minimized or even nullified if eaten improperly.

The Power Eating Program can teach you how to circulate your energy so you will receive the good, natural, and balancing forces of the universe and expel the negative, toxic, and imbalanced forces. Nothing can harm you as much as food, yet nothing can heal you more effectively than food. Eating is so primal an act that it is typically overlooked as a healing and transforming tool. To its credit, the macrobiotic movement has greatly awakened a public consciousness about the power of food.

We each choose what we want for our lives. With the Power Eating Program, you may derive the maximum benefits from the foods you choose to eat. As you begin to take more care with your choice of foods, eating manner, breathing, exercise, and quiet contemplation, and as you practice directing your energies, you will direct your life more swiftly to where you really want to go.

> *The mouth is the place to exercise our freedom, through breathing, talking, chanting, eating, and drinking. To manage the mouth properly is to manage your life properly.*
>
> Michio Kushi

SET YOUR GOALS

Before you eat, decide what you want out of life, out of your environment, and out of your food. Choose one or more of the following statements that are true about your goals, or create your own.

- I want to become totally healthy.
- I want to achieve my ideal weight.
- I want to become more confident and assertive.
- I want to become more calm and patient.
- I want to develop greater spiritual awareness.
- I want to experience more satisfying sex.
- I want to learn more quickly and thoroughly.
- I want to chew each mouthful _____ times.
- I want _____.

Now change the words, "I want to _____...." to "I am." Visualize yourself as you want to be. The more vivid your mental picture, the more powerful your results. Read this statement before every meal, as well as throughout the day. Develop a consciousness in your thinking and speaking. When we say the affirmation before and during our meals, the statement is "recorded" in the food and remains in you as long as the food is with you. Whatever we say and affirm tends to manifest in our life.

REALIZE WHY YOU EAT

The following seven reasons for eating are valuable to reflect upon as you become motivated to eat. They are all "right." Develop an awareness of your motivation for eating. Discover if the reason you are eating is:

1. **Mechanical:** A spontaneous response to hunger with no thought about the quality or effects of food. "I am hungry. I will eat anything. I could eat a horse."

2. **Sensory:** Eating for the taste, texture, odor, visual appeal of the food. "I eat this food because it tastes delicious. The food looks so pretty. I love creamy food."

3. **Sentimental:** Eating motivated by emotions, memories, or romance. "I eat this food because it reminds me of childhood, my homeland, the ethnic foods I loved. I want cookies and milk before bed."

4. **Intellectual:** Influenced by diet experts, scientists. "I eat this food because the book says to eat it. These foods are low in calories and high in vitamins."

5. **Social:** Eating with a consciousness for the earth and all people, with empathy for others. As Gandhi said, "I eat simply so that others may simply eat." "I eat food which supports the earth and can feed everyone."

6. **Ideological:** Eating according to a religious discipline or spiritual teaching, for development and transformation. "I eat the food of my spiritual beliefs, exercising discipline and care with eating."

7. **Supreme:** A freedom of eating with a foundation of deep wisdom and understanding of self and others, awareness of

all seven levels. "I eat to support my dream. I know the power of food. I eat to live, not live to eat."

(Based on George Ohsawa's Seven Levels of Judgement.)

A person should eat only when he has a natural desire for food, and not an indulgent desire. He who desires to preserve his physical condition should not eat before his stomach is purged of the previous food.

Code of Jewish Law

Dine with little, sup with less: Do better still, sleep supperless. Eat few suppers and you'll need few medicines.

Ben Franklin, vegetarian
Poor Richard's Almanac

ESTABLISH A SCHEDULE OF EATING

The Power Eating Program will clarify all aspects of optimum eating including the question of *when*. What, why, and how we do something are profoundly influenced by our timing. When you wake up, do you stumble into your kitchen to drink a stimulating beverage and gulp a quick breakfast? Consider your current habits. Do you rely only on food to give you an energy boost to begin your day? Do you have your largest meal at 9:00 at night?

Have you found your optimum eating schedule? While it is good to eat when you are hungry, some of us are hungry at times that may not be healthy for our digestion, such as late at night or constantly throughout the day. A student told me he ate only one meal a day ... all day long. I know it is fashionable to dine at 8:00 in the evening and stay up late. The Power Eating Program is about health, not fashion.

Ideally, the stomach should be empty before we add more food to our digestive system. For best results, allow five hours between meals. This will help the digestive organs to function well and prevent fatigue, indigestion, gas, or cramps. Three hours

13

is the minimum time we should wait between meals. Some people with hypoglycemia may need to eat every two hours in small amounts until they achieve health. If you eat three times a day, the best hours to eat are 7:00 a.m., 12:00 noon, and 6:00 p.m. Those having two meals a day may want to eat between 9:00 a.m. and 10:00 a.m., then again between 4:00 p.m. and 5:00 p.m.

My teachers, Michio and Aveline Kushi, present a dynamic macrobiotic educational program at The Kushi Institute Beckett Center, where healthful beverages are offered with a nourishing 8:00 a.m. breakfast. Lunch is eaten at 12:00 noon and the evening meal is eaten at 5:30 p.m. The Vega Study Center in Oroville, California, created by two wonderful macrobiotic teachers, Herman and Cornelia Aihara, serves early morning teas and soothing beverages, brunch at 11:00 a.m., and dinner at 5:30 p.m.

EXERCISE BEFORE EATING

Enjoyable, mild exercise is a health-giving activity at nearly any time, and especially preceding your meal. You might choose a session of Dō-In self-massage, three to five minutes on the rebounder, yoga stretches, or deep breathing. You need enough movement to get your oxygen and energy flowing without becoming over-stimulated or excited. The increased oxygen in your cells will help you digest and assimilate your food. Consequently, you will need to eat less. In answer to the eternal argument: "Which should I pay more attention to, exercise or diet?," I suggest attending to both — well and with consciousness.

At times we need a series of quick, easy stretches to get out the kinks before we eat. A few suggestions are listed below. These could not be more simple yet they stimulate your circulation and increase the oxygen flow in your blood to prepare you for the optimum eating experience. Enjoy these exercises seated before eating. As you perform each exercise, be sure to inhale through the nose and exhale through the mouth.

Lino's Simple Before-Meal Exercises

1. Sit comfortably with a straight posture. Look forward. Extend one arm to the ceiling while inhaling a deep breath. Exhale as you bring your arm down. Emphasize the exhalation. Repeat three to seven times, alternating each arm.

2. Stretch both arms slowly to the ceiling looking upward. Inhale and hold your breath. Bring your chin slightly inward. This will straighten your spine. Imagine that a string is attached to the top of your head, pulling you upward. Exhale as you slowly lower your arms to your side. Repeat three to seven times.

3. Inhale deeply and hold the breath. With your spine straight, exhale as you lower your head to the left shoulder. Inhale as you bring your head up, front and center. Exhale and allow your head to lower backwards. Inhale up again. Exhale and lower your head to the right shoulder. Repeat three to seven times.

4. Rub the palms of your hands together until you feel the warmth. Place your hands on your kidneys (lower back). Rotate your body around, inhaling while rotating backward and exhaling forward. Emphasize the exhalation. Repeat three to seven times.

5. Sit with your feet flat on the floor and in a straight posture. Inhale and place your right hand on your left knee. Exhale and twist to the left and look backward. Repeat to the right

side with your left hand on your right knee. Do this twist three to seven times on each side.

6. Place both hands on your thighs. Inhale and hold the breath. Exhale and bend forward. Inhale as you come up, exhale forward. Repeat three to seven times.

7. Inhale deeply and hold the breath. Relax your body. Exhale fully, allowing all tension to float away with the breath. (PEP contains an entire section on breathing in which you will learn the optimum breathing techniques.)

CLEANSE YOURSELF BEFORE EATING

If you have been out of the house all day, the best preparation for a meal is to take a shower and change into light, clean clothes. Get rid of the smells of the workplace and the vibrations of the streets. Remove the traces of cigarette smoke, car exhaust, and body odors.

If you have been at home and consider yourself clean, at least wash your face and your hands before the meal. You might use a warm face cloth such as those offered in Japanese restaurants. Cleansing purifies and stimulates your body and sets you in the right frame of mind to derive the greatest benefit from your meal.

ALIGN YOUR POSTURE

Once you have exercised and washed, relax your body and attain good posture. As in so many activities, your posture determines how well you do. When you eat, it is important to sit with a straight spine. Good posture enables you to more powerfully receive the energies surrounding you and to breathe more deeply.

To achieve a good posture at the table, simply raise your spine upward as though a cord were attached to the crown of your head. Stretch each arm up over your head several times. Tuck in your chin and buttocks without tension and begin to breathe deeply.

Directed breathing relaxes you before you go to table. It puts you in the proper state of mind.

James E. Loehr, Ph.D.
Jeffrey A. Migdow, M.D.
Take A Deep Breath

For the power of God's angels enters into you with the living food which the Lord gives you from his royal table. And when you eat, have above you the angel of air, and below you the angel of water. Breathe long and deeply at all your meals, that the angel of air may bless your repasts.

Jesus
The Essene Gospel of Peace

BREATHE DEEPLY AND SLOWLY

The Power Eating Program teaches you how to eat, which includes the importance and technique of proper breathing while you eat. In our stressed lifestyle, we have forgotten how to breathe! Air is our most essential element. We can live only a few minutes without it. The act of breathing, while automatic, can, with consciousness, become a powerful health practice. *The Journal of the American Medical Association* has published research showing that deep, slow breathing is an effective element in stress management. We all know how a deep breath can calm us.

Many cultures view the breath as the spirit. In fact, the root of the English word for "spirit" is "breath." The Yogi Prana, or Universal Energy, is synonymous with "breath." In Hebrew, "breath of life" can be translated "spirit of life." Our English word "inspire" is defined as "to breathe in, to infuse with spirit." Deep abdominal breaths are most effective for bringing in the oxygen we need to live. Babies naturally breathe this way. Sit or lie still for a few moments and notice where you are breathing. Is it from the chest or from the abdomen?

If you are breathing abdominally, your abdomen will move outward with each inhalation, and inward with each exhalation. Emphasize the out breath (exhalation) to rid your body of toxic air. Practice abdominal breathing throughout the day, especially at mealtimes.

Breathing well will increase the oxygenation of your blood. If your blood is oxygenated well, you will transmute your food better and assimilate and utilize the energy in it more effectively. Therefore, you will feel more satisfied with your meal.

Another tremendous benefit of conscious breathing during eating is the increased oxygen it supplies the brain, which uses up to 50 percent of all the oxygen our bodies take in. Better breathing creates clearer thinking. Our bodies are really quite a lot like machines. For optimum performance, we must use all the elements of matter and energy simultaneously.

Think of your new breathing technique as a means of balancing your eating, much like the workings of an automobile engine. The carburetor of your car mixes fuel with air to produce energy and power. Similarly, your body needs the proper balance of air and food to function efficiently. If the carburetor is clogged or maladjusted and too much gasoline mixes with too little air, the engine will cough and sputter, and the car will shake, then stall. You go nowhere. If this occurs in an airplane, you will force land or crash. Cars and airplanes are much less delicate than your body. Proper breathing while eating will create better "engine efficiency" and greater energy.

James E. Loehr, Ph.D. and Jeffrey A. Migdow, M.D., write in their book, *Take a Deep Breath*, "Slow, deep, rhythmic breathing triggers the release of endorphins. Breathing technique helps you digest food during main meals as well as temper appetite, and you will enjoy the meal more."

The best "fuel" for humans is whole grain because they are complex-carbohydrates which are high in fiber, low in fat, and nutritionally balanced. Whole grains help stabilize the glucose in your blood. Chewing these grains while breathing properly will give you more energy.

Ancient cultures knew this. The Chinese calligraphy for energy "Chi" combines the characters for "rice" and "breath." If your blood is clogged with fatty foods, the oxygen is unable to mix well in your cells. Consider your diet, your energy, your performance. Is it time for a tune-up?

TUNE IN TO UNIVERSAL ENERGY

Power, Life Force, vitality, electricity, vibration, Chi, Ki, Prana are all names for ENERGY. Used often in everyday conversation, energy has many meanings, from movement (kinetic), to electricity (power), gasoline (fuel), to Universal Energy (Divine Life Force). Whatever the meaning, somehow we know energy is good. We all want plenty of it.

Energy is the force of nature that flows through all things visible and invisible in the universe. Einstein taught us that energy can be neither created nor destroyed. It is eternal. The ancient Chinese called this energy "Chi," the Japanese word is "Ki." The yogis of India named it "Prana." In the West, this all-intelligent power is called "Universal Energy" and to some it is God. Different languages, the same idea.

Throughout history, enlightened people worldwide have experienced tremendous amounts of energy. These yogis and masters have been receptive, open, conscious, and blissful. Anyone can potentially develop such an evolved state, yet most of us remain blocked, caught up in everyday troubles and pain, too busy to see, hear, or feel the energy that is within us waiting to be awakened.

Dr. Bernie Siegel, surgeon, author, and teacher, writes in his book, *Love, Medicine and Miracles*:

> I think of God as the same healing force—an intelligent, loving energy or light in each person's life. Even scientists are now telling us that energy has intelligence.

In order to develop energy within, let us observe those who have achieved high levels of that "light," the enlightened. One commonality among the enlightened is that they fasted, as chronicled in accounts of Jesus and Buddha. These masters also meditated, spending long periods of time in prayer and contemplation, quietly listening, communicating with the Life Force that flowed through them. We each have the potential to experience the power of Universal Energy in our lives.

Are you thinking that you wouldn't know Universal Energy if it hit you on the head? Think again, or better yet, stop thinking so much! You experience Universal Energy any time you feel the warmth of your body, the rhythm of your pulse, or the freshness of a spring shower. You know it as attraction and repulsion, growth and death, pleasure and pain, and darkness and light. You know it as life.

*Everything on this earth has a balancing point
and in man this finds its place in the hara, the
place from which his vitality originates. If an
object's balancing point is close to the ground,
it is stable and cannot easily be knocked over.
Similarly, when a man's consciousness is centered in the hara, he feels very stable. At the
same time he feels abounding energy.*

Shizuko Yamamoto
Barefoot Shiatsu

DIRECT YOUR ENERGY

I often give a demonstration in my seminars. I stand and ask
someone to stand behind me and lift me up. Usually I am able
to be lifted very easily. Then I ask to be lifted again. The second
time it is always more difficult, as if I weigh an additional 30
or 40 pounds.

The first time I am lifted, I concentrate above my head and
direct my energy upward. This makes me light and easy to lift, like
a ballet dancer. The second time I focus downward on the *hara* -
the energy center located the width of three fingers below the navel.
I concentrate on my hara and breathe into my abdomen creating a
downward-flowing, more rooted strength. My partner has to pull
against my downward energy and seemingly heavier weight.

This simple demonstration dramatically illustrates the effect
of energy on matter. My energy was following my focus. We all
do this all the time. However, we usually lack consciousness in
directing our focus, allowing our energy to roam at random like
an untamed electrical current. I encourage you to direct your
energy with consciousness. As Thomas Edison channeled electricity, we too may direct our power toward greater enlightenment.

As all martial arts teach, if you "think from your hara," you will be more centered and will have more power than if you think solely with your head. Before meals and during exercise, it is best to focus your energy in your hara. During meals this focus should be in your mouth. If you watch television or read while eating, the energy will go to whatever you concentrate on, so you could say that much of the energy you receive from the food will go into the television or book.

If you stand while eating, most of your energy will go to your legs and you will derive much less benefit from the meal. If you sit, or better yet, kneel down, the energy will center more effectively. If your eating posture is correct and you properly focus your awareness, you will tremendously increase the transformation of food into energy.

RECHARGE YOUR ENERGY

Your body receives downward-moving energy from the heavens (Heaven Energy) through the spiral at the crown of your head. Conversely, the Earth Force spirals up through the soles of your feet and your genital area, then meets and connects with the Heaven Energy. Our entire body is a miraculous, living receptor and generator of electromagnetic energy. Seven *chakras*, or energy centers, gather and disperse this Life Force throughout your body. The amount we absorb and utilize depends upon our condition and how we live our lives.

The Heaven and Earth energies meet in our mouths while we chew. Heaven's downward-flowing, contractive energy forms the *uvula*, the cone-shaped piece of tissue hanging down at the back of your throat. The earth's expanding energy spirals up through your tongue. As your food is chewed, the uvula and the tongue charge the food, and a transformation of energy takes place. The more we chew, the more we "get a charge out of life."

Correct posture is very important, especially when one is self-reflecting. Both the seiza posture and full lotus posture are very good for this purpose. One should sit completely relaxed, as though planted between heaven and earth ... and the spine should be held straight. If the body slumps forward or backward, the natural flow of energy is impeded and the nervous system is stressed.

Shizuko Yamamoto
Barefoot Shiatsu

ESTABLISH AN EFFECTIVE EATING POSITION

There are many reasons for eating, many goals for eating, and many positions in which to eat. The choice is yours. After years of research, I have concluded that the optimum position for eating is the *seiza* (say za) position, which resembles the position of meditation and prayer. (See Illustration.) Seiza may not be the position you choose daily, but it is the ideal one. I encourage you to experiment and to notice your energy with each position.

The worst position for eating is walking. This is because the energy leaves the digestive tract and circulates all over the body. The second worst position for eating is standing because energy goes to the legs. Better than standing is, of course, sitting while you eat. Sitting gathers the energy to the hara, the digestive center, stomach, and intestines. There are several effective sitting positions. One is in a chair with legs down, in the typical manner with straight posture. Another position some people like is crossing their legs Indian- ("lotus") style. Again, in my opinion, the optimum eating position is the seiza.

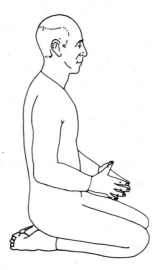

SEIZA POSITION

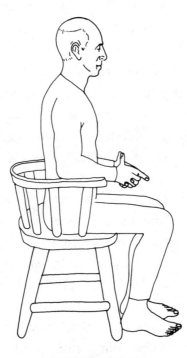

SEATED MEDITATION

More About Seiza

There is a science behind seiza, the optimum eating position. Kneeling is practical, not mystical. Observe the seiza position. The center of gravity is in the hara. If you eat in this position, you will eat less food and derive more energy from it simply because the energy is not dispersed through your limbs. You are concentrating your energy in the hara and connecting more closely with the earth, which produces the food you eat.

As you eat, kneel as if you were about to begin a meditation or prayer. Keep the back straight and tuck the buttocks in. Feel the energy moving down to the hara. Feel yourself becoming more centered. Eating can be as balancing as a meditation. According to the *Essene Gospel of Peace*, Jesus taught his followers, "Eat slowly, as it were a prayer you make to the Lord. For I tell you truly, the power of God enters into you, if you eat in this manner at His table."

Therefore, two or three times a day, the art of eating and the art of meditating can become *one*, increasing the power of food. As with meditation, acquiring a soft cushion on which to sit, and perhaps placing another one under your knees, will help make the position more comfortable. You may wish to obtain a seiza bench to help you be more at ease.

When you kneel to meditate, pray, or eat, keep your big toes crossed behind you and hold your fingers together loosely in your lap. This will enhance the flow of energy from one side of the body to the other and balance the energy in both the right and left sides of the brain. You can place your fingers in a meditating position. (Illustration A.) Or you may wish to link your fingers. (Illustration B.) A third hand position is one that Michio Kushi teaches. Put your pointing (index) fingers together facing downward with your thumbs together. (Illustration C.)

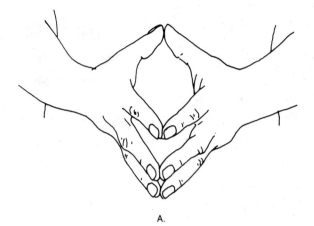

A.

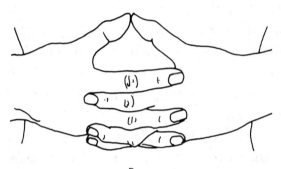

B.

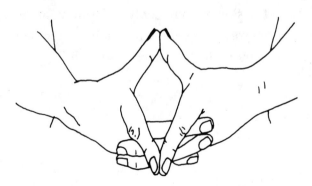

C.

This position relaxes your shoulders. According to Oriental medical theory, the lung meridian (energy channel) flows through the thumbs. When you connect your thumbs, you complete a circuit that strengthens your lungs and thus your breath.

In addition, the large intestine meridian flows through the index fingers. Energy from the lungs goes to the large intestines, affecting your entire digestive tract. When the feet touch each other, and one hand touches the other hand, the energy circulates throughout the body. When such a posture is adopted while eating, *a powerful energy cycle is formed.*

The energy will flow down each leg, across the toes and back up your other leg, then the energy moves down each arm, across from one hand to the other and up your other arm. The energy flow then circulates from one side of your body to the other and meets at the hara. The body is now aligned to receive and circulate maximum energy at its fullest. *You will literally be recharging yourself as you eat!*

Choose any position you prefer, from sitting in a chair to sitting crosslegged or kneeling on a floor cushion. Whatever position you choose, remember to be aware of your posture and the energy flow. Sit straight. Concentrate on your mouth or on your hara. Breathe slowly and deeply. As you maintain correct posture and visualize energy flowing from your mouth to the hara, the energy you build can be very powerful.

Every minute is meditation. To develop your meditative powers, be attentive to the world around you. In this way, little by little, you will come to understand your true relationship to the universe.

Shizuko Yamamoto
Barefoot Shiatsu

TRY MEDITATING AT MEALTIMES

There are many places now throughout the world where eating is practiced as a meditation. For example, Beckett, Massachusetts is the beautiful mountain setting of The Kushi Institute's Spiritual Development Seminars. Michio and Aveline Kushi teach profound ancient wisdom as students experience a daily practice of conscious living.

Jane Quincannon attended the Kushi Institute Spiritual Development Seminar and reported in *Return To Paradise* about her powerful experience of conscious eating. "We were served simple, delicious meals, which we chewed 150 times per mouthful using a special meditation technique taught by Michio. Many of us were amazed at how little food we needed and how our vitality rose during the seminar. I learned many other lessons just from the eating, about excess, emptiness, greed, arrogance, clarity, and gratitude."

When I visited the Tassahara Zen Center in Carmel, California we ate in the meditation hall in absolute silence. In such an environment, a small quantity of food is quite satisfying. At Kripalu Center in Lenox, Massachusetts, one has meals in the "Dining Chapel" where silence is observed. On each table is a small sign which reads, "Silence is Golden. Share it with a friend." At the Aihara's Vega Institute in California, a silent chewing area is provided at mealtimes.

In silence, O dear one, eat without haste. With peace, delight, and one-pointedness, thoroughly chew your food. Don't eat merely for the pleasure of taste.

Swami Muktananda
Reflections of the Self

CREATE QUIET MEALTIMES

As a boy on my grandfather's farm in Yugoslavia, we had many people at our main noon meal. Besides our family, we were often joined by up to two dozen field workers. After everyone was served, hardly a word was spoken. The meal lasted an hour and a half, after which we rested under the tree or in the haystack until 3:00 p.m. Then we resumed work until sundown and ate our evening meal in the same manner.

Talking while eating tends to send the energy from the mouth to your throat or brain, creating a separation of energy in the body and disrupting the digestion process. We receive much less energy from the food when we expend the energy by talking. An Italian saying, "Quando si mangia non si parla" means, "Whenever you eat, don't talk." Many cultures have adopted similar practices.

I have observed that people who talk while eating often need larger quantities of food and experience more frequent indigestion. Therefore, it is best to practice silence while eating or to speak as seldom as possible between bites. Turn off your television, telephone, or loud radio as you eat. Many people find that soft music is very relaxing at mealtimes.

If you must talk socially while eating, discuss pleasant topics. Avoid any negative topics of conversation because you will charge the food with negative thoughts and as your food gets digested, the negative energy will go inside you. Charge your food with thoughts of strength, joy, and appreciation and the same will become you.

Make mealtimes relaxing. Even the best quality food can be indigestible if you are tense or disturbed when you eat it. Create a quiet and relaxing time for meals. If you have children and meal times are a little hectic, or if you are exposed to unsupportive attitudes about your food when you eat, change your meal time for a while, and eat by yourself.

Bill Tara
The Joy of Life

Don't be discouraged if you find relaxation procedures hard at first. Relaxation and meditation are perhaps especially difficult for Americans. Our constant mental diet of advertising, noise, violence, and media stimulation makes it very difficult to endure even a few minutes of inactivity and quiet ... the quiet can be threatening.

Bernie Siegel, M.D.
Love, Medicine, and Miracles

LEARN TO RELAX!

In this modern, high-tech age, it seems we have to learn how to breathe, to eat, and now to relax. Our culture is so fast-paced and competitive that stress, both a cause and symptom of disease, is epidemic in America. In the old days, folks sat on their porches in the evening, chatting, sewing ... relaxing! The days began at dawn and were filled with physical activities from chopping wood to tending the garden. Jogging was unnecessary, unless you had to run after the plow, or chase your sweetheart through a field. By dusk, almost everyone was ready for bed. Forget sleeping pills or tranquilizers!

Nostalgia is fun, but few of us want to return to the old days. However, we must make changes to bring a more lasting tranquility into our modern lives. Relaxation has been proven to improve digestion, reduce high blood pressure, and strengthen the immune system. The Prana, or Life Force, can flow much better in a relaxed body. James E. Loehr, Ph.D. and Jeffrey A. Migdow, M.D. in their book, *Take A Deep Breath,* offer more excellent reasons for relaxing while eating:

> The glands in your mouth produce two kinds of saliva. When the diner is relaxed and ready to eat, the parotid glands produce saliva that contains digestive enzymes and is watery; it easily digests food being chewed. Under stress, however, the sublingual glands exude a thick saliva that is devoid of digestive enzymes. Clearly, relaxing before a meal is the first step toward ease of digestion. By timing chews with breath in a meditative manner, a relaxed mood can be preserved throughout the entire meal.

Before eating each meal, before you begin another day, learn to relax. Attend yoga or meditation classes which teach relaxation techniques. Discuss your anxiety with a counselor. Learn to let go of stress. In this world, relaxation has become another essential discipline for health and transformation ... *so learn to relax!*

A GUIDED RELAXATION...

You have exercised, cleansed yourself, achieved good posture in a comfortable seated or kneeling position, and begun deep abdominal breathing. No need to talk, argue, or debate. You experience just being with your body in all its magnificent spirit. Now you feel your body relaxing, shedding the stress of the day with each exhalation. Breathe. Close your eyes. Visualize a lovely scene of nature. Experience the freshness and the peace.

Straighten your spine. Tuck in your buttocks without tension. Rub the palms of your hands together as you breathe deeply, until you feel the heat of energy between your hands. This begins the flow of energy throughout your body. Relax your arms with your hands clasped comfortably in your lap. Sit still for a few minutes and breathe abdominally, at least seven times, the slower and deeper the better. This type of breathing will center and relax you and keep the energy moving.

Close your eyes and send loving thoughts from the top of your head throughout your body, downward, filling your arms, your chest and abdomen, down your legs and into your feet. Continue until your whole body is relaxed. Send the loving energy to all organs or areas that needs special healing. Now extend that love outward to your family, friends, city, continent, as it flows over the entire earth and into the limitless heaven ... and back into you.

INCLUDE GRATITUDE IN YOUR ATTITUDE

We have discussed how to prepare for eating. We have talked about stretching, cleansing, breathing, posture, and relaxation. Now, before we begin to eat, we should give thanks. Does it really make a difference? Think about how you feel when a friend expresses love and gratitude to you. This is exactly how the food feels.

Food is alive. Food is not a dead, inert, or unmoving object. Food is a blessing from the earth. When food is unappreciated or wasted, I often become extremely upset. It is as though a dear friend were criticized or thrown away. Today Americans have such abundance that people have lost their reverence for food. The practice of fasting creates a profound awareness of the blessing of food.

Talk to food as if it were alive because it is alive. You can speak aloud or silently to the food as though it were a small tape recorder on which you record your words, thoughts, and emotions. Tell your food, "Please go inside my body. Help to heal and energize me, speed me up or slow me down, help balance me." Direct your food's energy to best nourish your special needs.

The food can sense your gratitude and will respond to you. Think of the different foods as little genies or spirits on the plate that will enter your body and do magical things for you. Realize how fortunate we are to have food. Express your gratitude to Nature, God, the Universe, to all the people who bring the food to you, and to the food itself. Only then, after you have given thanks, should you begin to eat.

LINO'S MEALTIME PRAYER

Thank you, Universe, for giving us life, for inspiring us and guiding us. Thank you for our parents, mates, and friends who share our lives. We deeply thank you for the food we are about to receive. We thank everyone who brought the food to us, from the farmer who grew it, to those who deliver it to us. We especially thank the cook who prepared this food and now serves it to us. May this food go inside our bodies and help make us healthier, better balanced, and happier. May it purify us, so that we become better human beings with more awareness, who make this world more healthy, peaceful, and happy. Amen.

CHOOSE HEALTHY EATING UTENSILS

In 1972 I lived in Providence, Rhode Island where I established a macrobiotic center and restaurant with an associate. One day we went to a close-out sale of a Chinese restaurant. My friend was delighted to buy antique wooden chopsticks. After the sale, we returned to our restaurant to eat lunch.

My friend started to eat his meal with the chopsticks he had bought that morning. Suddenly, he began to eat very fast. Over time we noticed that every time he used that particular set of chopsticks he tended to eat faster than normal. It was as if he were picking up a vibration from the chopsticks. He could not explain this phenomenon.

Whoever used the chopsticks also ate quite rapidly and left his or her energy on the utensils. Your fork, chopsticks, bowl, spoon, and everything you use absorb a vibration from the person who used the object before you. As you use the utensil or dish, you, in turn, will pick up the same vibration.

I eat as slowly as I can. My favorite eating utensils seem to help me because over time, they have absorbed my vibration. If I feel like eating fast because I have a lot to do that day, they slow me down. This may surprise you. Yet, you would agree that happy people can make you feel happy. Nervous people can make you feel nervous. Calm people can make you feel calm. So why shouldn't eating utensils transmit energy from the vibration of the person who used them?

Why do some people use wooden chopsticks rather than metal forks? Because energy flows better through organic materials such as wood. These natural materials transmit a strong flow of energy from nature to your food and into you. So avoid using metal utensils whenever possible. Instead, try to use cookware,

38

utensils, and dishes made of organic material such as wood, clay, or ceramic.

SET YOUR TABLE TO SET YOUR MOOD

Serving food in a beautiful manner is a high art all over the world. We are as nourished by our food's appearance as we are by its nutritional or energetic value. We can help balance our conditions by the ways we present our meals. With consciousness, we can arrange and serve our food to enhance our pleasure. When we are served beautiful, simple meals, we feel loved and cared for.

Consciousness in eating is no better illustrated than in the Japanese Tea Ceremony. When taking part in a tea ceremony one does not answer phone calls, conduct business or do things unrelated to the ceremony itself. The ceremony becomes a joyous discipline of total focus, like poetry. Every item in the tea ceremony is immaculate, beautiful, cherished, and often quite valuable.

Eating is the act of creating your body, your very life. What more important act do we perform daily? What more profound way do we honor and love ourselves? It is the primary way to "gain" energy as almost everything else we do causes us to "spend" the energy we have. Just as in the tea ceremony, everything connected with preparing and eating our meals should be of the finest quality we can afford. Our energy, our enjoyment, indeed our very lives will reflect that consciousness.

Color can be a healing influence, nowhere more profoundly than in our table settings. Red makes us feel warm and stimulated. Earthy tones of brown, gold, and russet bring us warmth and stability. Blues, greens, and pastels cool and calm us. White is neutral. Choose colors for your table that complement the season and the effect you desire.

In the winter, warming colors along with more rustic materials of pottery and wood balance the cold climate. Cool colors and smooth textures such as glass and porcelain are appropriate for the hot summer months. Color influences can be carried over to napkins, table cloths, and vases. Chinese emperors used to change their household colors every season.

We bring nature indoors through our food, and we can add more touches of nature to our table. First, clean your dining table well. If it is used as a workspace, clean it before each meal. Put away distracting papers that you may be tempted to read as you eat. From your yard, find greenery, flowers, tree branches, leaves, pine cones, even colorful stones that are pleasing or whimsical to the eye.

As you eat, you may want to look out at a lovely scene in nature, or at a beautiful flower, branch of a tree, or plant. In the evening, perhaps you may want to light a candle on which you can meditate. It is proven that such visual scenes tend to put our minds in an alpha state where we are more receptive to healing and positive energy. These touches need not cost much, yet their value to you will be priceless.

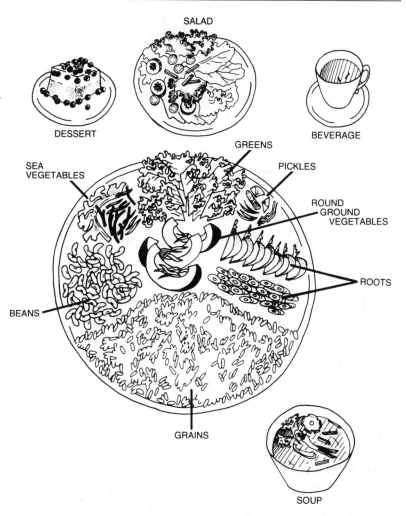

SALAD

DESSERT

BEVERAGE

GREENS

SEA VEGETABLES

PICKLES

ROUND GROUND VEGETABLES

ROOTS

BEANS

GRAINS

SOUP

ARRANGE YOUR FOOD FOR BEST RESULTS

Arrange the food on your plate as if you were painting a picture, and just as from a work of art, its energy will enter through your eyes, making your whole spirit and body feel better. Food should look good and taste good to be good for you. Learn to enjoy your food with all your senses: sight, taste, touch, smell, and even the sound it makes in your mouth.

Eating your food in an orderly way becomes easier when you arrange your food in a conscious, proper way on your plate. The grain should be on the side of the plate nearest you, the beans to the left of the grain. If your meal's protein is fish, place it to the left of the grain where you generally put the beans. Arrange the root vegetables to the right of the grain. Sea vegetables are placed on the left above the beans, pickles on the right above the root vegetables and leafy greens on the top of the plate directly across from the grains. (See Illustration p. 41.)

While this is an optimum arrangement, you may alter the design to emphasize the effect you want the food to produce. Serving food becomes both an art and a science as you control the physical and sensorial impact of the presentation. The addition of special side dishes and condiments lends variety and enhances the total eating experience.

EAT YOUR FOOD IN THE PROPER SEQUENCE

Throughout the world, people know intuitively that we should start our meals with a cup or bowl of soup. In some countries where the climate is warm or the individuals are hot due to a high-protein diet, the meal is started with a cool salad or a cold drink. This is why Americans, who eat per capita 150 pounds of meat a year, prefer their cocktails and salads before the meal.

I suggest eating the soup first. The soup is usually slightly salty. Eaten at the beginning of the meal, soup stimulates the flow of saliva and enzymes in the mouth. This helps to predigest carbohydrates and release the stomach's digestive juices, including hydrochloric acid (HCl), which digests protein and fat. Soup may be finished before eating your main course or it may be sipped throughout the meal as your beverage.

Eating your meal sequentially from foods that are more condensed to foods that are more expanded will promote the best digestion and elimination. After the soup, take between a teaspoon and a tablespoon of whole grain. Place your eating utensil down on the table. Chew your food very well. Swallow. Then take a spoonful of beans or fish (it is generally best to avoid eating both at the same meal). Put your utensil down. Chew well and swallow. Return to the grain. Put down your utensil as you chew. Next, take a bite of root vegetables. Lay down your utensil. Chew well. Alternate bites of grain with portions of each kind of food in this sequence:

1. Grain	6. Round, ground vegetables
2. Bean	7. Grain
3. Grain	8. Sea Vegetables
4. Roots	9. Grain
5. Grain	10. Leafy greens

Continue this optimum eating cycle, alternating your grain between each spoonful of other food. Remember to place your utensil down between each bite and to breathe deeply as you chew. These techniques will help you eat more slowly and receive maximum benefits from your meal.

Toward the end of the meal, take a piece of pickle as needed or desired to aid digestion. If bread and salad are served, they should be eaten after you have finished the main course. Finally, eat desserts or sweets at the end of the meal with your beverage. People who tend to produce flatulence (gas) should wait at least 15 minutes after the main course before eating dessert.

Grain should be eaten throughout the meal to promote an orderly assimilation of different foods. Grain's high fiber also assists the peristalic movement through the intestines. This way of eating will virtually eliminate chronic constipation, which in my opinion is a pre-cancerous condition. Eating whole grains in the proper way is the single most powerful action you can take toward good health.

This sequence represents eating according to energetic laws, from heavy, concentrated foods that need more enzymes and digestive juices—to lighter, more expansive foods—alternating both with balanced grain energy. In cultures throughout the world, meals have traditionally been eaten in this order.

The Japanese words "kami" (chew) and "kamu" (to chew) mean God or Divine Spirit. Chewing in the original Japanese meaning is "to develop ourselves, to reach to the Universal Spirit."

Chewing is one of the fundamental ways of expressing our freedom. Everyone can chew according to their own desire. The more you chew, the greater the possibility that you will develop your consciousness as well as improve your day to day life.

Michio Kushi

*And chew well your food with your teeth, that it
become water, and that the angel of water turn
it into blood in your body.*

Jesus
The Essene Gospel of Peace

*Since the digestive process begins with grinding
the food with the teeth and by mixing it with the
juice of the saliva, one should not swallow any
food without masticating it well, because it will
overtax the stomach and make digestion difficult.*

The Code of Jewish Law

*Chew well! Anyone who is sick or who wants to
be beautiful and intelligent must chew well before
anything else. Chewing well increases not only
your physical health, but also your related mental
and spiritual clarity. Judgement improves.*

Herman Aihara
Basic Macrobiotics

CHEW:
CONSCIOUSNESS FOR HOW TO
EAT WISELY

Throughout my years of studying Oriental medicine and macrobiotics, I practiced the art of chewing. I knew chewing was a simple
act—the simplest, yet done with consciousness it can be phenomen-
ally powerful. Macrobiotics teaches that chewing is a primary factor
in health and transformation. In my research I found recommendations for chewing well from yogis, athletic physicians, Jesus,
Gandhi, Muktananda, nutritionists, beauty experts, and a British
Prime Minister. I chewed on it all … and agreed!

I still had many questions. "How can one gain energy only

from water?" "Why is it beneficial to continue chewing after the food has become liquid?" Although my students and I experienced remarkable improvements from chewing, I continued to search for more information.

Noboru Muramoto, my longtime sensei (teacher), provided me with the missing link. In his book, *Natural Immunity, Insights on Diet and AIDS*, Sensei Muramoto provides research and insights into the causes of and solutions to all diseases, especially AIDS. He devotes an entire chapter to chewing. His book inspired me with new information, and most of all with his enthusiasm about chewing. When Sensei Muramoto visited me in Florida, I noticed how well he chewed his food.

According to *Natural Immunity*, scientific studies by Dr. Tomozaburo Ogata of the School of Medicine at the University of Tokyo indicate that chewing strengthens our immune system and promotes rejuvenation. The salivary glands produce enzymes that begin digesting carbohydrates in the mouth, a process that is vital to vegetarians. Also, chewing stimulates the release of parotin hormones which encourage the thymus to create T-cells, the protectors of our immune system. Parotin hormones are released by the parotid glands, located on each side of our jaw behind our ears.

All foods, especially carbohydrates, begin the process of digestion in the mouth. Chewing enables the digestive enzyme ptyalin, found in the saliva, to mix well with carbohydrates. Ptyalin breaks down the carbohydrates, beginning the dynamic process of transforming food into energy. In addition, vegetables must be chewed well to break down the tough cellulose that surrounds the plant's nutritive core. The stomach cannot digest carbohydrates.

It is imperative to chew grains well. Poorly chewed grains

cannot break down properly and thus the nutrients, protein, and starches will not be separated from the fiber. If grains are swallowed without proper chewing, the pancreatic enzymes will be unable to break down the food into its basic components. In this case, the grains will only be partially absorbed by the intestines.

At this stage, the unabsorbed, partially digested food particles move to the large intestines, where intestinal bacteria ferments them. Fermentation produces excessive carbon dioxide, and sometimes, methane (if there is an odor.) The result: gas and bloat.

If you don't want to chew, *any diet*, especially one high in complex carbohydrates, will fail to produce the desired effect and may create gas, heaviness, discomfort and sluggishness. Poorly digested food can sometimes produce mental and emotional side effects such as irritability, moodiness, and anger.

Dr. Arthur L. Kaslow, a California physician specializing in nutritional medicine, notes a distinct correlation between his patients' chewing habits and their digestive functions. "Chewing is an essential part of a good digestive program. In our extensive two week stool examination, we have discovered that too many patients don't chew well. These people usually experience gas, bowel and digestive problems. We live in a time of fast food, fast eating, and fast chewing. We must reorganize our priorities in order to regain our health."

The human body is designed to eat grains and vegetables. Dr. Robert Haas, famed athletic nutritionist and President of The American College of Sports Nutrition, counsels some of humankind's best physical specimens. Dr. Haas advises in his book *Eat to Win, The Sports Nutrition Bible*, "Chew every mouthful of food until it is liquified in your mouth." Professional athletes throughout the world are adopting the powerful diet composed of whole grains and vegetables. Perhaps we can learn from the animal kingdom. The strongest animals in the world and those with the most endurance eat vegetation which they chew very well.

Carnivorous animals have teeth with which to tear. Plant-eating herbivores have teeth with which to grind. We are omnivores who can tear and grind our food. Of our 32 teeth, only four are sharp, tearing tools. As Jane Brody, nutritionist for *The New York Times*, reports in *Jane Brody's Nutrition Book*, "Our teeth are more like those of herbivores than of flesh eaters. Our front teeth are large and sharp, good for biting, our canines are small, our molars are flattened and our jaws are mobile for grinding food."

Human intestines are four times as long as those of carnivorous animals, which means our digestive system has plenty of time to digest high-fiber plant foods. However, decaying animal food needs to exit the body quickly and because our intestines are so long, animal foods tend to remain in humans too long, creating putrefaction, excess wastes and fats, and as research has shown, cancer. Countries with low per-capita meat consumption have virtually no colon cancer. As humans, we have the choice of putrefying or purifying our bodies.

We can eat a high-protein diet and take the consequences with cholesterol, fats, chemicals, and toxins or we can be more vegetarian and enjoy the physical, mental, emotional, and spiritual benefits it has to offer. As John Robbins states in his passionate and powerful book, *Diet For A New America:*

> Thousands of impeccably conducted modern research studies now reveal that the traditional assumptions regarding our need for meats, dairy products, and eggs have been in error. In fact it is an excess of these very foods, which had once

been thought to be the foundations of good eating habits, that is responsible for the epidemics of heart disease, cancer, osteoporosis, and many other diseases of our time.

If we choose to eat more grains and vegetables, the foods that sustain life on earth for all, *we must chew our food*. The strongest animals in the world such as the ox, bull, elephant, and buffalo are plant eaters who chew their food very well. If you do not chew well you will not digest your food and will tend to overeat. The more you chew, the more powerfully you will transform your food into energy. If you eat macrobiotically to heal yourself and you fail to chew properly and enough times, the diet will be far less effective or it may not work at all.

I know of no better analogy for chewing than building a fire. Try it yourself. Build a pile of paper and put three or four thick logs on top. Light the paper and see what happens. The paper will flare up, the logs will be blackened and the fire will go out. No matter how dry the wood is or how good the wood is, the chances are 1,000 to 1 that the wood will not burn.

Now try chopping the wood very finely, as thin as kindling. Try again. What happens this time? It doesn't matter how hard the wood is, if you chop it finely, you will be able to start the fire and generate heat and energy. All boy scouts know this.

If you chew your food finely enough you will release the energy absorbed by the plants from the sun, the earth, the moon, and the stars. As you chew these pure vegetarian foods, the universal energy is released to help provide the power you need to ignite a healthier, more vital life. Perhaps this is what Lord Krishna, the highest Indian deity, refers to in the *Bhagavad Gita*: "I live within you in the form of the digestive fire." Let us practice what boy scouts and sages have always known.

I have made it a rule to give every tooth of mine a chance, and when I eat, to chew every bite thirty-two times. To this rule I owe much of my success in life.

William Gladstone
19th Century British Prime Minister

How Much Should I Chew?

Horace Fletcher was perhaps the greatest chewing advocate the world has ever known. In poor health, obese, with chronic indigestion and fatigue, Fletcher, an American college professor, traveled to Europe at the turn of the century where he learned of Prime Minister Gladstone's chewing recommendations.

Fletcher adopted Gladstone's "rule" of chewing each bite thirty-two times and even increased the chews to fifty. He also ate only when calm and rested. This new regime was a huge success! Fletcher quickly regained his health and became a renowned athlete and world-record-breaking weight lifter. This revolutionary thinker wrote about and taught his eating theory, known internationally as "Fletcherism."

Unfortunately, Horace Fletcher did not know enough about nutrition and the importance of whole grains. He recommended that students spit out the fiber of the food they chewed. Consequently, his followers failed to receive sufficient nourishment and Fletcherism got "spit out" as well. However, George Ohsawa, the pioneer of modern macrobiotics, studied Fletcherism and adapted the chewing techniques for macrobiotics.

In my opinion, 50 times a mouthful as recommended by the standard macrobiotic diet is really the minimum number one should chew each mouthful. If you want to get your digestive "fire" really burning and produce strong energy, then you must chew at least 100 times.

However, if you have an ailment or are seeking above-average energy, you should chew 100-150 times. To help recover from serious illness and degenerative diseases or if you are taking drugs or radiation therapy, you will need to chew each mouthful 150-200 times. If you are so sick that the doctors have given up on you, chew each mouthful 200 times or more. Aveline Kushi often recommends that people with serious conditions chew 200 to 300 times or more.

Gandhi said, "Chew your drink and drink your food." Chew even your liquids, and chew your food until it becomes liquid before you swallow. Once you have chewed 150 times, there is really nothing left to chew. The food will be entirely liquified and mixed with your saliva. That way, the food is predigested in the mouth and the intestines will not be required to work as hard.

NOBORU MURAMOTO'S CHEWING RECOMMENDATIONS

The following are estimates for the time needed for chewing at each meal:

— For healthy people, about fifty times, which means about thirty minutes per meal; if talking time is included, you need an hour or more as you wish.

— If you have some health problems, you should chew each bite a hundred times or more; this will take about an hour just for chewing.

— If you are seriously ill, try to chew two hundred times or more and take at least two hours for your meal. This amount of chewing is needed in order for parotin to be produced from the saliva and absorbed into your bloodstream.

(Reprinted from *Natural Immunity, Insights on Diet and AIDS*.)

Students at my PEP Seminars and I have discovered that after eating and chewing one hour we are usually quite satisfied and rarely need to eat more. I realize that for most of you, chewing well and taking more time with eating will be a major change in your life. Yet, it may be the change you need. Try it!

At the 1989 Miso Soup Bowl, the annual Macrobiotic Foundation of Florida winter seminar, I met a Chinese man who remarked that chewing is an ancient Chinese technique for rejuvenation. He told me about a man in Hong Kong who teaches Chinese rejuvenation techniques, including chewing. One afternoon session costs $1,000! *You can chew for free!*

Saliva heals. Have you noticed how a dog will lick a wound? If you have a small cut, saliva speeds up the healing process. *The Journal of the American Dental Association*, May 1988, contains a research study indicating that saliva contains an antibacterial substance that prevents the AIDS virus from infecting white blood cells. Saliva is a powerful and essential element in the transformation of food into energy.

Chewing is the spark that lights your inner fire. Throughout my life, I have seen my theory of chewing proven time after time. In all my experiences in war refugee camps, the army, the restaurant business and in macrobiotic teaching, I have observed that people who chew more are healthier, stronger, and happier.

While my father was in a German concentration camp, he sometimes chewed his food 300 times per mouthful. Other prisoners who did the same were able to survive the experience as he did. Those who wolfed down their food, finishing everything in a few minutes, died sooner. It is very difficult for some people to chew well. But if you can do it you can live on half or less of a normal meal. I saw this happen again and again. This is one of the most profound and practical things I can teach you.

At What Rate Should We Eat?

If I am eating alone, I can chew very well. I can chew even better in the company of people who chew well. If I eat with people who are not willing or able to chew, they affect the way I eat. We are each affected by our environment and by the people around us. For maximum benefits from your food, choose a peaceful, supportive setting in which to eat.

Throughout my life, my glands have been over-active. If you eat with me, you will notice that although I chew more than most people, I often finish before others. This is because I chew faster. I am constantly aware of this and try to chew more slowly. The faster we eat, the more hyperactive we become. A cycle begins that influences our entire life. However, we can change our energy patterns.

If you are slow and lethargic, and wish to revitalize your metabolism, consciously speed up your chewing pattern. If you want to be calmer and slow down your metabolism, then purposely slow down the speed of your chewing. You can set the stage with background music and lighting. Bright lights and peppy music speed up the rate of eating. Soft lighting and slow music will create a more tranquil pace of chewing.

Remember, the rate at which you chew your food affects the energy in your entire body. Chew consciously, with awareness, as you adapt your chewing for your daily needs. The important thing is that you chew your food well. I realize that the discipline of chewing requires great patience. Yet once people experience the miraculous results, they feel it is worth the effort.

Chewing is most important in macrobiotics.
You have no teeth in your stomach nor in your
intestines. So you must chew in your mouth, 50 times
per mouthful, at least. The more you chew,
the quicker you will master our philosophy of
longevity and rejuvenation. If you have no time to
chew, or if you are so busy in your business
that you cannot taste quietly your food and drink,
you have no qualification to step into this
Macrobiotic diet. In reality, good
chewing of well-balanced food is the greatest
ceremony of creating Life.

George Ohsawa
Practical Guide to
Far Eastern Macrobiotic Medicine

Nature will castigate those who don't masticate.

Horace Fletcher
The ABC of Nutrition

MASTICATION CAN BE FUN

Necessity certainly is the mother of invention. My students have created some remarkable methods to make chewing more fun and effective. I'll share some with you. Let me know ways *you* invent to chew more!

1. **Say a positive affirmation in rhythm to your chews.** One of my favorites is, "Every day in every way I feel better and better." Count how many beats to your affirmation and repeat it in your mind as you chew.

2. **Count only up to ten.** Ten times! Keep track on your fingers.

3. **Time how long it takes to chew the number of times you desire.** As you take each mouthful, set a timer (I prefer using a silent hourglass) then relax and let your mind flow until you hear the tone or see that time is up.

ADVANCED CHEWING TECHNIQUES

In the beginning when you train yourself to chew, you may find that old habits die hard. The tendency is to swallow after 20-30 chews. When that happens, consciously stop chewing for a few seconds and push the food forward with your tongue. Then start again. At about 50-80 chews, you may have a lot of saliva, especially if you took a large portion. If this happens, swallow some, and next time take a smaller bite. At 150 chews, most people find they can chew indefinitely because the reflexes become automatic and under control.

Chew in a spiral motion for best results. In the beginning it may feel strange as most people chew up and down. You can train yourself better if you push the food with your tongue left to right from one side of the mouth to the other every 25 bites or so. The whole experience becomes more and more pleasant (even if it seems monotonous) until one begins to feel calm and relaxed.

An additional technique that I have found powerful is to keep my eyes half-closed or closed as I repeat my affirmation. I visualize what I would like to manifest in my life. This technique registers my affirmation in my subconscious, thus helping my dreams and desires become reality.

Sometimes I have the feeling that I am chewing with my whole body and feel heat all over. It is then that I experience the ultimate "high" of eating. This usually happens to me at about 200 chews. The experience is best described as a high feeling of well being, a glowing, tingling sensation all over my body that feels intoxicating. After you experience this sensation, you may become hooked on chewing purely for the invigorating feeling. I call this feeling the "Body Energy Glow."

The Body Energy Glow is like many other pleasurable physical sensations. For instance, athletes often get a "rush" when they run full stride. Lovers experience a high when they are near their beloved. Others feel this energy flow when they are joyfully involved in singing, dancing, chanting, or playing. Some of you will experience the chewing glow very soon. Others may find it takes more time for the body's energy to unblock and flow freely. Practicing PEP will better enable you to fully feel life's multitudes of pleasures.

Brown rice is the food that gives the best high. In my opinion it is because the rice changes into natural sugar more readily and contains the most "ki" or life energy. Truly, brown rice is the king of grain.

After a meal you should feel light, energetic and buoyant, as though you were floating in the air, feeling very, very good, happy to be alive and grateful for everything you have, especially the food you have just eaten. I am sure that chewing increases the endorphins in the brain and body, and makes you feel so good that you believe you can handle anything. You may become energized and optimistic, as though you are in love or deeply inspired by nature. Chewing is an exercise that makes you feel in love with your body and all of life.

When I began the Macrobiotic Way of Life to heal my cancer, I announced to my family that I was going to chew my food 50 times a mouthful. I received great support from my husband and children. Though they ate 'regular' food, we had our meals together and they helped me stay on my program. My son, Jeffrey, would watch me eating and remind me if I did not chew enough. 'You only chewed 35 times, Mom'!, he would say. With all my chewing, I was still at the table long after my family finished eating. One day Jeffrey said, 'Mom, why don't you begin eating a half hour before we do so we can all finish together?' This made me aware of just how much I had changed. I was taking more time and care with my eating. It paid off. The macrobiotic way of life, especially my new diet and way of eating, saved my life. I have completely recovered.

Elaine Nussbaum
Nutritionist
Author, *Recovery*

*As Lino's dentist, I feel like I am working in the
pit crew of the world's greatest chewer.*
James Harrison, D.D.S.
Lake Worth, Florida

SINK YOUR TEETH INTO THIS

In my counseling, I always look at my client's teeth to determine
how well he or she will be able to chew. If your teeth are in poor
shape or are missing, it is critical to fix them as soon as possible.
Get all gaps filled in so you can chew your best. It will be one of
the most important investments you can make, so give it top priority!

If you must wait to have your teeth corrected, purée your
food with a hand grinder. There are two basic kinds, a "hand
mill" grinder, usually made of stainless steel, and a small plastic
baby-food mill. Avoid using a blender because its electrical vibration is disruptive to your energy and the air that is mixed into
the food may cause gas and indigestion. Even if you purée your
food, always mix it well with your saliva.

We all need to eat our vegetables. Yet, if crisp vegetables
are difficult for you to chew, avoid the habit of cooking them all
until they are very soft. This can deplete their nutritive and
energetic value. It is essential to cook food in a variety of ways.
If chewing is difficult for you now, cook your vegetables in many
different methods, with an emphasis on a light, crisp style. Then
purée the vegetables. Remember, though, nothing really replaces
the act of chewing.

Only the chewing motion stimulates the release of the ptyalin
enzyme and the parotin hormone, both vital digestive and rejuvenating elements awaiting release into your body. Therefore,
take good care of your teeth. They are your tools of the trade—

trading sickness for health.

EAT YOUR FOOD AT THE PROPER TEMPERATURE

Most food should be eaten warm, at least at room temperature, particularly if you are a "cool type" of person. You are a "cool type" if (a) you dislike cold weather; (b) your hands and feet get cold easily; and (c) you sneeze often and catch colds frequently. You are a "hot type" if (a) you love cold weather; (b) your feet and hands are always warm; and (c) you perspire easily.

If you have excessive body heat or if the weather is hot, then cool foods, such as salads will refresh you. Icy cold foods may produce cramps, or even paralysis in the stomach. When your stomach becomes cold from icy foods and beverages, the gastric juices stop flowing, creating indigestion.

People who desire cold foods are generally those who consume an excessive quantity of animal protein, which produces a lot of heat. They have a high internal heat and eat icy foods to cool off. However, this can be dangerous. These people actually need to eat a better-balanced diet to regulate their body temperature.

When you eat, never eat unto fullness. Give heed to how much you have eaten when your body is sated, and always eat less by a third.

Jesus
The Essene Gospel of Peace

Never eat until you are full. Overeating causes excess, which, if it is not discharged, will cause imbalance as more is taken in than is given off. Overeating brings the blood to the lower digestive regions of the body. It therefore takes blood away from the brain. As a consequence, clarity of thought is sacrificed through overindulgence. In order to respond accurately to the challenges of life, the mind must be alert. A person with a healthy appetite who eats only to 80-percent capacity can become very successful—his health will be secure and his direction will be clear.

Shizuko Yamamoto
Barefoot Shiatsu

CHOOSE THE RIGHT QUANTITY OF FOOD

We have now discussed *what* to eat and *how* to eat. The next question is, *how much should we eat?* If your body is functioning really well, your stomach should be about the size of your own fist and ideally this is the amount we should eat. The best way to measure this amount of food is to fill up a bowl or measuring cup with water. Put your fist inside up to your wrist. You can then measure how much water you displace. It is considerable.

If you are really healthy, one fist-sized amount of food is how much you should need at each meal. One fist-size is approximately the size of an average soup bowl, and coincidentally, the size of your stomach. Although one such serving should contain all the nourishment you need, very few people are actually satisfied with that small amount of food.

For most of us, two fist-sized meals is usually the minimum, but most of us eat about three fist-sized portions of food per meal, or more. Many of us have enlarged stomachs. Therefore, if you eat until your stomach is three-quarters full, your stomach will slowly shrink to a smaller, more healthy size and you will begin to be satisfied with less food. Remember, don't bite off more than you can chew!

Now that the natural foods movement is well underway in this country and in Europe, I have recently become interested in other important aspects of healthy eating. They are the amount of food that we eat and the way we eat.

My interest was stimulated by the works of Mizuno Nanbuko, the most well known and respected physiognomist in Japan. Several hundred years ago, Nanbuko wrote that the quantity of food we eat determines our health and destiny. In the opening chapter of his book, soon to be translated into English as Food Governs Destiny, Nanbuko writes, "Food is the essence of life, and everything we do is governed by how we eat. We should always hold food in the deepest respect. Food is really of the greatest importance."

After reading Nanbuko, it dawned on me that I had not paid enough attention to the amounts of food I was eating. I discovered that even if we ate the best quality of foods, eating too much of them would spoil the benefits we received.

I also realized that trying to control the amount we eat can be very difficult. The key, of course, is chewing. Recently I tried chewing each mouthful 300 times and was surprised at the energy and awareness it generated. These experiences taught me the true meaning of digestion.

Chewing helps us to be modest and appreciate the foods we are given. Without chewing well, information about diet and health is of little value.

Aveline Kushi

Want to learn how to eat a lot? Here it is: Eat a little. That way, you'll be around long enough to eat a lot.

Anthony Robbins
Unlimited Power

Do not overeat. Most persons die as a result of greediness and of ignorance of right dietary habits.

Sri Yogananda

I saw few die of hunger; of eating, 100,000.

Benjamin Franklin
Poor Richard's Almanac

How Much Food Is Too Much?

Imagine your body fully satisfied, vibrating with life energy, perfectly nourished, relaxed yet keenly aware. Do you believe you can achieve that state? Visualizing is the first step. The Power Eating Program can start you on your path to nutritional satisfaction and balanced weight. With the commitment to consciously eat the healthiest foods on the planet, you cannot fail to achieve the transformation you seek. You can be satisfied and eat smaller amounts!

Overeating is a crime against your body. Some people who are overweight *do not overeat*, and others who are slender *do overeat*. Practicing PEP's principles can help reduce body fat as well as obsessive food cravings. Observe how various people eat. Study the quantity and quality of their food choices.

Quantity changes quality. Your body can digest only so much food. The rest is deposited as fat or toxins. When these fats and toxins come out, they manifest as pimples, cysts, boils, and crusts. When blocked inside they form internal cysts, tumors, and fatty layers around your organs. Excess food creates stagnation of the Life Force Energy.

There are many causes of overeating, physiological and psychological. Some diet experts say, "It's all in the mind," others proclaim, "It's all in the body." The truth is that the mind and body function as one. If you are overeating, learn to heal your mental attitudes, fears, and personal traumas through counseling, support groups, and workshops. At the same time, change the way you treat your body. Through proper practice of the Power Eating Program, you can begin to do both.

The cause of all disease is arrogance.
George Ohsawa

Stagnation is the cause of all arrogance.
Michio Kushi

How Will PEP Help Me To Eat Less?

The three major ways the Power Eating Program can balance your consumption of foods are:

1. **Better Absorption:** When healthy food is chewed well, your digestive tract will absorb its nutrients. You are often hungry because you are undernourished, either by the consumption of devitalized, processed food, or because you are gulping large, unchewed mouthfuls into your stomach. *Many people are over-fed and under-nourished.* You don't have to be one of them!

2. **More Satisfaction:** The sole act of chewing has a powerfully calming, satisfying effect on people. You must try it to understand what I am saying. When I chew very well, I am quite content with half my usual amount of food. Please try it!

3. **Deeper Relaxation:** Tense, hyperactive people often overeat. Eating has a relaxing effect on the body. Eating is a primal need, yet like all "needs," it can be redirected into constructive life patterns through conscious relaxation and meditation, as I teach in this book.

A TOAST TO GOOD HEALTH

I am not wishy-washy about liquids. I see too many people who have symptoms of liquid imbalance. Are you drowning your kidneys? Those valiant little organs the size of your ears courageously attempt to filter all the soft drinks, hard liquor, and fruit juice guzzled in this society. Americans love beverages "on the rocks." And that's just about where this nation's health is heading.

If your diet includes animal foods like fish, chicken, meat, cheese, and eggs, you will need more liquids to balance their high protein, sodium, and toxicity. If you are frequently thirsty, seriously look at your protein and salt intake. Read labels. Become aware. If you are eating a grain and vegetable diet, you will need fewer liquids, since vegetables and cooked grains have abundant water content. Cooked whole grains have up to 70 percent water and vegetables contain 85-95 percent water.

Drink your beverages *after* your meal, as they will dilute vital digestive enzymes. Drink when you are thirsty. Chew your beverage well (25-50 times) for best results. This will mix the liquid with your saliva and bring it to body temperature. Notice when your body is hungry and thirsty. As you become more balanced, listen to your intuition regarding eating. Your body will tell you how much to eat and how much to drink.

PRACTICE PEP AFTER EATING, TOO

When you have finished eating, remain at the table for a few minutes. Continue to breathe deeply. Express loving gratitude to the food for becoming part of you. Sit and drink your tea and discuss pleasant topics. Keep in mind that the energy of your words and thoughts deeply affects you, especially during and after mealtimes.

Rest quietly at the table for at least ten minutes, preferably twenty minutes, to allow the food to begin its transformation into energy. If you get up immediately after eating, the energy will go to the moving parts of your body. Retain the energy in the digestive tract for as long as possible to maximize the full absorption of the total eating experience.

After this short relaxation, it is fine to get up and move around. That is the time to wash the dishes and clean up the dining area. Move slowly and calmly. It is important to continue breathing deeply. This oxygenation of the blood, along with tranquil movements, will ensure better digestion.

TAKE AN AFTER-MEAL STROLL

One of the best ways to help your body assimilate food and complete digestion is to take a walk after the meal. It doesn't have to be a long walk. Just a stroll for ten minutes is often adequate, and half an hour is even better. If you work in an office building, going outdoors for a walk after lunch to get fresh air will improve digestion.

Walking helps you breathe more deeply. When you breathe, you burn your food better and release more energy from the same amount of food. The National Institute of Health in Bethesda, Maryland, states, "Walking is the most efficient form of exercise-

and the only one you can safely follow all the years of your life." Ideally we should walk 30-45 minutes after every meal, and especially after dinner.

AVOID SLEEPING AFTER EATING

After you have eaten, the very worst thing you can do for your body is to go to sleep. After lunch, wait at least one hour before taking a nap. Following your evening meal, wait at least three hours before going to sleep; four hours is better, and five hours is best. Ideally, your stomach should be completely empty before meals and when you go to sleep. Much of the body's regeneration and healing occurs while sleeping, but only if the stomach is empty. So, if you go to bed at 11:00 p.m., finish your evening meal by 7:00 p.m.

Michio Kushi teaches that "eating immediately before going to bed has the similar effect as eating animal foods. It creates improper digestion, gas formation, emotional heaviness and general fatigue." What I understand by that is that the energy of the body gets congested and blocked, producing stagnation and deep imbalances. Therefore the body cannot heal, unblock, recharge, and balance itself. You will then likely wake up in the morning feeling sluggish, cranky, or clouded after sleeping poorly or for too long. Incidentally, the less you eat, the less sleep you need to recharge yourself.

PEP STEP BY STEP

Here is a condensed version of PEP:

1. Exercise, practice Dō-In, yoga, ect..
2. Take bath, shower, or at least wash your face and hands.
3. Turn off the television, radio, and telephone.
4. Find a clean, quiet place to eat.
5. Light a candle or play soft music if desired.
6. Perform table exercises if you haven't exercised.
7. Sit with a straight spine.
8. Express gratitude or read an affirmation.
9. Begin conscious breathing.
10. Place a bite of food in your mouth.
11. Place eating utensil down.
12. Begin chewing and deep breathing.
13. Concentrate in your mouth or hara.
14. Look at the food or other attractive object.
15. Place your hand with fingers touching.
16. After eating, say a word of gratitude.
17. Rest and/or talk for 10-15 minutes.
18. Take an after-meal stroll.

sticky deposits create energy blockages and therefore the energy inside becomes stagnated.

However, if you follow the principles of PEP and eat healthful foods that balance your unique condition, you will naturally establish your best weight. Even cellulite can disappear. You will first lose the excess weight, then the fats around the internal organs. Your energy and Life Force will begin to flow more powerfully throughout your body.

6. **Creates Clearer Thinking and Better Mental Health:** The Japanese word for chewing means "good understanding." In Oriental medicine, the brain and the small intestines (hara area) are connected energetically. The condition of the intestines greatly affects our thinking capabilities, thus the terms "meathead," "egghead," and "fathead." If we eat less and chew more, our thinking becomes clearer and our brain functions better, especially if we breathe deeply while eating. The majority of the oxygen we take in goes to our nervous system and to our brain. In addition, the oxygen helps digest our food. The combination of less food and more oxygen creates a greater flow of energy. More importantly, this combination helps your food to change into glucose, which helps provide your body with energy.

7. **Enhances Results From Any Diet:** Carbohydrates are digested in the mouth with the help of the ptyalin enzymes in your saliva. By practicing the Power Eating Program, including eating relaxed meals and chewing thoroughly, we increase the benefits of any diet. Of course, the healthier the diet, such as macrobiotics, the better the results.

8. **Saves Money:** As you practice the Power Eating Program, you will become more satisfied with less food, and therefore

will spend less money on your groceries. In addition, your health will improve, thus reducing costly medical bills. Americans spend over $200 billion a year on health care. Notice what people eat and how they eat. Know that there is a connection between their eating habits and their health.

9. **Reduces Cravings for Sweets:** People who chew very little often need sweets with meals. Those who chew complex-carbohydrates well are able to experience the inherent sweet taste of these foods and frequently are able to decrease their craving for sweets. It is especially important for people with hypoglycemia or diabetes and related disorders of the pancreas and spleen, (which largely control the blood sugar), to chew very well - 150 times or more. These organs process sugars. The more we chew, the sweeter the food becomes. This sweet flavor, along with relaxed mealtimes, will help satisfy a need for relaxing food (sweets).

10. **Improves the Taste of Food:** Food, especially grain, becomes sweeter as it is chewed. Many people who practice PEP discover they develop a greater and greater appreciation for simple meals. They simply become more satisfied with less, as they absorb more! Herman Aihara has this to say about chewing for improvement of taste: "Chew 50 to 100 times, which also makes the food delicious. Chewing gives you the real taste of food, enabling you to distinguish between good food and bad; real food tastes better the more you chew."

11. **Reduces Flatulence:** Quite a lot of people suffer from intestinal gas. There are two kinds of flatulence. One type of gas has no odor and occurs because of inadequate chewing and overeating. If you chew your foods calmly and quietly, you will eat less and reduce flatulence. Odorous flatulence occurs

in people who have poor digestion due to an unhealthy diet, poor food combining, improperly cooked foods, or inadequate chewing. PEP provides clear solutions to overeating, indigestion, improper food combining, and improper chewing.

12. **Encourages Relaxation:** Many people are tense and have a lot of stress. The more calm your mealtimes are, the more peaceful the energy you take into your body will be. This will carry over throughout your day. When chewing is done as a meditation, a mealtime becomes prayer-like; a powerful, calming, and healing experience you may enjoy two or three times a day.

13. **Reduces Bad Breath:** Breath odors come from several sources. Most people who have chronic bad breath overeat or eat too often. Before they finish digesting one meal they eat another. They snack and nibble between meals. Their daily routine might be breakfast, then a coffee break, lunch, a snack, dinner, then another snack before bed. Three meals a day should be sufficient if you eat properly. Many people are satisfied with two meals a day. Remember, we have the choice of putrefying or purifying our digestive systems. A healthy digestive system generally signifies a healthy body and mind. An old folk saying is: *Sweet breath means a sweet disposition.*

14. **Activates Glands:** The Power Eating Program will affect your entire endocrine gland system. Chewing activates all the glands, from the pituitary and thyroid to the pancreas, spleen, and gonads. The sex organs become more balanced. The gland that undergoes the most change is the thymus gland, which produces T-cells necessary for a healthy im-

mune system. According to *The American Medical Dictionary*, research indicates that the parotin hormone, which is excreted during chewing, increases T-cell production. Chewing well is vital for people with AIDS or with any degenerative disease.

15. **Creates a More Alkaline Condition in the Body:** A healthy body is balanced on the alkaline side. Yet, because of eating foods that tend to produce large amounts of acid, including meat and sugar (*the per capita U.S. consumption of each is over 150 pounds a year!*), most Americans are suffering from an over-acid condition. Chewing creates a more alkaline condition in your body because the saliva is alkaline and as it mixes with the food it alkalizes the food you swallow. Even grains can create an acidic condition if not chewed well. This is yet more evidence to support good chewing.

16. **Helps Heal Ulcers:** Chewing increases the *quantity* as well as the *quality* of saliva, which is healing for all tissue, internal and external. I often suggest to people with stomach or digestive disorders to hold an umeboshi (pickled plum) pit or clean pebble in the mouth to stimulate the production of saliva. Saliva is a natural alkaline medicine which, when swallowed, neutralizes excess acidity in the stomach, and helps relieve ulcers.

17. **Prevents Death by Choking:** The National Safety Council reports that 2,500 people die every year in the U.S. from choking on food. Choking, or "Cafe Coronary" for which the Heimlich maneuver was developed, is one of the five main causes of accidental death in the United States, occuring when people swallow a piece of food that is too large. Careful eating can eliminate many of these needless deaths. If you

can teach your children to chew well, you may help to save their lives.

18. **Creates Stronger Teeth and Gums:** Chewing stimulates the flow of blood and energy to the teeth and gums because you use them more.

19. **Reduces Food Cravings:** Many people have strange cravings. They don't know why. If you chew a healthy diet well, you will probably discover that your craving for unhealthy foods will diminish. Many people become more satisfied with the foods they eat. Since I have been chewing really well I have less desire for animal food such as fish. My cravings for desserts and fruits diminishes as my chewing increases. This has been a miracle for me.

20. **Improves Creativity:** Calm, meditative eating and chewing helps you become a calmer, clearer channel for inspiration. Consider the "starving artists" who produce their best work in poverty with little food. Small quantities of food allow a stronger flow of ki, chi, or prana through the body. Excess food creates stagnation of the body, mind, and creative energy channels. Inspiration has as its root word "breath." Oxygen can most freely flow in a body clear of stagnation and excess fats. Creativity on all levels increases when we are attuned with nature, through conscious living.

21. **Enhances Marriages and Relationships:** Michio Kushi writes in *The Book of Macrobiotics*, "Without eating whole balanced meals together, there can be no biological, psychological, and social unity, which is the essence of the family. When family members eat in separate ways and at separate times, dissatisfaction and division spread. Though

there may be other contributing factors, the fundamental reason for the increase of conflicts, arguments, separation, and divorce among married people and the disintegration of the modern family is a decline of the home-cooked family meal."

The family that eats calm, balanced meals together will become more centered, stronger, and more relaxed. They will most likely have a better chance of staying together. How did your family eat their meals today? All at different times, perhaps at different locations, on the run, between appointments, late at night? Such chaotic eating creates stress and blocks the internal organs, creating stagnant emotional responses. Balanced meals, eaten in a calm, pleasant manner and eaten by your whole family together, will produce greater harmony both within your body and within your family.

Most of us know what it is like to be around irritable people. Our health profoundly affects our behavior and emotional responses. An old term used to describe an angry person is "liverish." In Oriental medicine it is taught that the condition of the liver greatly influences the expression of anger. A balanced diet, eaten in the optimum manner, can have a powerful effect on our body as well as our emotional well-being. Our relationships will reflect the health of our body. Conversely, our daily interactions have a bearing on our health.

If you have children, feed them one to two hours before the adults. It is easier to chew when small children are well fed and away from the table. Children are generally hungry for dinner around 4:30 to 5:00 p.m. If they eat then, they can play for two hours before bed. This will give them time to digest their food. Avoid putting a child to bed directly after eating. As I have stated before, this is unhealthy for anyone. Children usually do not want to go to bed after eating because the food gives them energy and they want to use it up.

22. **Promotes Rejuvenation:** Chewing has rejuvenating benefits. The Hunza society of the Himilayas are known for their longevity and practice of chewing. Extensive research on rejuvenation has been conducted by Dr. Tomozaburo Ogata, a professor at the School of Medicine at the University of Tokyo.

According to Noboru Muramoto's book, *Natural Immunity*, Dr. Ogata discovered that chewing revitalizes the body because it activates the parotid glands, located on each side of our jaw behind our ears. The more we chew, the more active the gland becomes, secreting the hormone parotin. If one chews too few times, the hormone is swallowed and destroyed in the stomach. Chewing your food well causes the parotin hormone to become absorbed through the lymph system. The hormone renews the cells, affecting the entire endocrine gland system and rejuvenating the whole body.

Dr. Ogata observed that people do not *want* to chew, so he extracted the parotin hormone from cow's saliva and injected it into some patients. In a few months the participants looked ten years younger, but in time the effects diminished because the hormone is meant for cows, not humans. Each of us can chew and produce our own revitalizing hormones.

23. **Enhances Development of Psychic Powers:** With the adoption of a vegetarian diet, there is a purer energy flow in the body on all levels. When the diet is eaten properly, in a calm, meditative manner, with aligned posture and deep breathing, then powerful changes occur in the mental and spiritual channels. Stagnations disperse, allowing the energy

channels to open, inspiration to flow, and intuition to clarify.

24. **Creates Greater Sexual Stamina and Vitality:** It is only logical that anything that increases energy and improves our health will also improve our sexual organs and our sex life! Impotence, infertility, nonorgasm and PMS are primarily the results of blocked energy and poor nutrition. The Power Eating Program teaches effective exercise, breathing, eating, chewing, and relaxation, which contribute to better circulation, vitality, stamina, and sexual satisfaction.

25. **Improves the Condition of All Organs:** PEP teaches how to improve your total health, whichever diet you choose. As you know by now, the diet I recommend is the grain-and vegetable-based macrobiotic diet eaten in the proper manner. In the June 1989 issue of *Macrobiotics Today*, Herman Aihara writes of the liver and chewing. "One of the reasons chewing is so important is that it will make us eat less. Then our liver will be healthy. This is the first step toward longevity and brilliant health. There is no real health without a good liver and there is no good liver without chewing well."

26. **Increases Efficiency:**

Taking time for chewing means you will take less time to accomplish things.

Michio Kushi

It seems the more I chew the more time I have! I accomplish tasks at a greater speed and efficiency. The clock becomes an ally.

Jane Quincannon

MY FIRST MACROBIOTIC PEP SEMINAR

The beautiful Smokey Mountains were the setting of the first macrobiotic seminar in which I taught the Power Eating Program and in which all the students practiced it. Greg and Michelle Samples of the Macrobiotic Center in Knoxville, Tennessee, organized the weekend retreat, held at the lovely Sterchi Lodge, situated at an altitude of 3,000 feet. Each day the fresh air was cleansed by a light spring shower. The temperature was ideal and invigorating, cool for early July.

People came to the seminar from Tennessee, Georgia, and North Carolina. Greg assisted me with teaching and counseling, while Michelle, with two cooking assistants, prepared three superb, tasty, and healthful meals each day. A choice of three macrobiotic diets was offered: a low-salt diet for pre-menstral women and persons with high blood pressure or salt sensitivity; a second diet to speed up metabolism and lose weight; and a standard macrobiotic diet that was balanced for general needs. Cooked and fresh fruits were available at all times for everyone.

I observed and evaluated the group carefully at dinner the first night. Five students seemed overweight by at least twenty pounds; six were definitely weak and needed stronger energy; and except for three, all chewed about ten times per bite. After dinner, during a personal evaluation session, eight students out of twenty-one said they felt overweight, eleven expressed feelings that they needed more energy, twenty craved sweets after every meal, and several said they never felt satisfied after eating.

Each day we did limbering exercises, and Dō-In self-massage. We also massaged each other lightly before each meal. At the table we read personal affirmations designed by each student. We encouraged each other to practice the PEP principles of good posture, slow, deep breathing, and quiet, relaxed attitudes. Before

83

and after each meal, we spoke a grace of thankfulness. We ate our meals in silence as we chewed very well. The atmosphere was extremely peaceful, centering, and nurturing.

After eating, we drank tea and discussed the day's experiences and personal questions. Students began to share their results with the macrobiotic diet and with PEP. After the first day everyone chewed over 150 times! Most had no sweet cravings and ate much less because they felt more satisfied with the food. Two students experienced Body Energy Glows, a warm, tingling sensation in the body.

At the last meal, twenty out of twenty-one students had no sweet cravings. This is desirable for people with the tendency to have hypoglycemia. Eleven students experienced the Body Energy Glow and we all ate less. Everybody felt more emotionally stable, mentally clear, and generally better. One person who was determined to experience the energy glow chewed each bite 400 times for an entire meal and achieved it!

The individual who got the most out of the seminar was a fellow who had progressive paralysis on the left side of his body spreading to the right side. When he came to the retreat he could barely walk. He had seen many doctors and specialists who were unable to diagnose the problem. It was not polio, M.S., or any other known disease. When the seminar was over, the student could walk more easily. We all hope that he will continue to eat and chew well to achieve full recovery.

For me, this mountain seminar was a remarkable experience. I can't help but think that miracles such as this don't just happen in concentration camps, but can happen at anyone's dinner table.

PEP SUCCESS STORIES

When my wife, Marquita, and I chew our food at least fifty times a mouthful, we experience the benefits of good digestion. This leads to a calm and peaceful relationship.

Warren Wepman
Attorney
Miami, Florida

For me, chewing is a discipline. When I concentrate on chewing each mouthful 100 to 200 times, I experience a rejuvenation in both body and mind. When I chew well, it takes me about one hour to eat, so realistically, I can't chew that thoroughly at every meal. When I don't chew each mouthful 200 times, I chew at least 50 times.

During my mealtimes I meditate and relax—something I have difficulty doing in my otherwise busy routine. When I chew well, my stomach feels satisfied and not bloated. At these times, I never feel that my body needs to take time off to digest the food. I'm ready to go, whether to a game of tennis, for a horseback ride, or to pursue a mental activity.

When I chew well, I eat less food. I've discovered that my body actually functions more effectively on little fuel. I experience more energy and stamina on a small amount of food that has been digested well in my mouth (chewed until the food becomes liquid), than when I stuff myself on a macrobiotic feast.

Also, I have noticed that the graying of my hair has slowed down to a crawl from its rapid pace of two years ago. That was when I first became conscious of chewing my drink and drinking my food. Several of my students have also reported the positive effects that chewing well has had on their lives.

Judy Paris, B.S. Physical Education
Lecturer, teacher, Vice-President
Midwest Macrobiotic Center
The Greater Cincinnati, Ohio Area

I first became aware of the importance of chewing when I heard Lino Stanchich at the 1988 Miso Soup Bowl Conference in Miami. I later participated in his PEP Seminar in the Tennessee Mountains where we practiced and studied the energy of chewing for an entire weekend. At Lino's retreat, I learned to incorporate walking in my daily regimen. I now take a walk each morning before I go to work and at night after my evening meal.

My new exercise routine, my deeper awareness at each meal, and my thorough chewing have been a revelation. My digestion and level of energy have improved greatly. I have been in the brokerage business for over twenty years. Lately, even my success in the stock market is markedly better. I'm looking forward to continued benefits from these new daily habits that are helping to change my life.

Stephen Cohen
Stockbroker
Atlanta, Georgia

I was in my last year of college—my last semester. For some reason, I couldn't remember the material I was studying. I would forget the information after a few days, and sometimes after a few hours. My head had ached for weeks. When I sat down to think about my health, I realized with horror that meat had crept back into my diet. In addition, I desperately wanted to end an unfulfilling relationship. I had no car, no job, and my only source of income, a rental property, was vacant. I felt my life was out of control.

For months I had wanted to visit the Macrobiotic Foundation of Florida. I felt that by taking control of my diet, perhaps I could begin to recreate my life. I went to the foundation where I met and talked with Lino Stanchich, the senior macrobiotic counselor. Lino was honest with me about my diet and suggested many changes in my food and its preparation.

Lino insisted that I cook food on a gas stove. I couldn't afford one, so he loaned me his camping stove. I was surprised that Lino stressed changes in other habits as well. Lino encouraged me to resolve my home situation, to sing and exercise daily, and to chew very well. He told me to chew each mouthful at least 100 times.

While chewing, I was to sit in a peaceful, quiet place and concentrate on the things I wanted to bring to myself, and focus on achieving positive changes in my life. Because Lino was so adamant, I immediately began to make the changes in my life and to practice the eating habits that he recommended. I especially concentrated on my chewing.

Changes started to happen! I found the courage to have an honest discussion with my partner. We both decided that a break in our relationship would be best for both of us. Two weeks later he sold me his car at an unbelievably low price. Soon after, I got a call from a woman who wanted to rent my home. She offered to fix it up, too!

My life had definitely taken a better turn. During this time, I noticed an ad at school from a major corporation looking for someone in my field. When I went to the interview, I discovered that I knew the head of the department. I was hired that day. A week or two after, I was also offered an assistantship at the university.

I firmly believe that the change in my diet, and especially my chewing, enabled me to redirect my life. I was able to quickly change my living situation. Improvements in my health, my attitude, and my life have steadily grown more positive.

My major change was four years ago. Today I am a gourmet natural foods chef working for a private company. I am studying acupuncture and also applying for my state nutritionist license. I own a new car and new house. My daughter attends a private school. I feel very happy and in control of my life. Many things have changed for me. There is one thing that will never change —I will always chew well!

Nedra Hiday
Gourmet Natural Foods Chef
Miami, Florida

A new philosophy, a way of life, is not given for nothing. It has to be paid dearly for and only acquired with much patience and great effort.

Fyodor Dostoyevsky

Health must be made by yourself. One who makes himself healthy knows the law of change. He can change sickness to health, sadness to joy, and enemy to friend. He is a free man.

George Ohsawa

MY GREAT LIFE JOURNEY

Macrobiotics means *macro*: great, *biotics*: life, and for me it has been just that, a great life of transformation. Through practicing macrobiotics I began to understand my body, my mind, my spirit and the power of nature. The macrobiotic principles of energy, natural living, and true personal responsibility changed me. For the first time I experienced full control over my life, my health, and my evolution as a human being. This knowledge gave me a freedom I had never felt before.

Based on ancient wisdom and refined by noted Japanese teachers, macrobiotics has become a vital international movement, a true blending of East and West. The macrobiotic way of life teaches that we are a part of nature, and the more we live according to natural laws, the healthier and happier we will be. The best way to become attuned with nature is to eat foods that are fresh, seasonal, organic, and local, chosen to balance our own unique conditions and needs.

Macrobiotics teaches us the profound effect food has on our physical, emotional, mental, sexual, and even spiritual well-being. We are deeply influenced by the foods we ate in the past,

89

for these are the foods that have created the very foundation of our being. Clearly, a balanced, natural diet enhances anyone's personal program of health.

According to The National Academy of Sciences, diet contributes to 60% of all illness. The American Cancer Society, which tells us, "A defense against cancer can be cooked up in your kitchen," suggests that we eat more high-fiber foods such as fruits, vegetables and whole grains. The macrobiotic diet includes all of these nutritionally sound foods.

"What we eat may affect our risk for several of the leading causes of death for Americans," U.S. Surgeon General C. Everett Koop states in his 1988 *U.S. Surgeon General's Report on Nutrition and Health*. Koop goes on to say, "Diseases of dietary excess and imbalance are among the leading causes of death in America." The Surgeon General joins the National Cancer Institute, the United States Senate, The American Cancer Society, and the National Academy of Sciences in recommending a diet containing more whole grains, vegetables, dried beans, and fruits.

The foundation of the macrobiotic diet is whole grains. Interestingly, the Far Eastern term for "peace" combines the two words "rice" and "mouth." Throughout history, these nutritious, natural, high-fiber grains have sustained mankind but they have recently been neglected in the Standard American Diet (SAD), pushed far into the background behind dairy foods, meat, and refined grains. As a result, the health of this nation's people and land has profoundly suffered.

Raising animals for food is destroying the earth and the health of its people. John Robbins, in his powerful book, *Diet For A New America,* has calculated that for each year that an individual eats a pure vegetarian diet, one acre of trees is saved. In the United States, an acre of trees is cut every five seconds.

Robbins states that the cause of most of the waste of the earth's natural resources is the American meat-based diet.

As Robbins teaches, our planet would have more than enough food to feed the 60 million people who starve to death each year if people ate the grains that are now fed to livestock and, if Americans reduced their intake of meat by only 10%, *everyone* would have enough to eat. We must unite as world citizens and change our diets. However, in order to absorb the grains and vegetables properly in our bodies, *we must learn how to eat them properly.* PEP will teach you how.

At first I ate the macrobiotic diet to feel better. Soon I discovered how right the diet was, not only for my health, but for the survival of our planet and its people. I was impressed by the common-sense logic of macrobiotics and I searched throughout New York City for more information. Twenty years ago, one of the primary macrobiotic resources in New York City was the Caldron, a small restaurant in Greenwich Village. I resigned from my managerial position and took a job in the Caldron's kitchen where I began to learn how to prepare macrobiotic foods. There I was, a European, eating brown rice and miso soup with chopsticks in America. It seemed crazy, *yet nothing had ever felt so right.*

Though my prior American diet had consisted primarily of heavy gourmet restaurant dinners and ethnic feasts, beginning the macrobiotic way of life was, for me, like putting a fish into water. I loved it. My entire body loved it too. In addition to eating whole grains, I began to eat a delicious variety of pasta, breads, beans, fish, vegetables, sea vegetables (these took a while to get accustomed to), salads, fruits, special condiments, and beverages.

I embarked on an intense study of macrobiotics with Michio and Aveline Kushi in Boston, as well as with Herman and Cornelia

Aihara, and Noboru Muramoto in California. These teachers were devoted students of George Ohsawa, the pioneer of modern-day macrobiotics. After fourteen years of dedicated macrobiotic study and practice, I passed the requirements for certification from the Kushi Institute and became a macrobiotic teacher and counselor.

During my years of counseling, I have known numerous people who experienced dramatic healing with the macrobiotic grain-based diet. Several became authors of excellent books about their recovery through macrobiotics. Among these moving testimonials are Dr. Anthony Sattilaro's *Recalled By Life, Recovery,* by Elaine Nussbaum, Virginia Brown's *Macrobiotic Miracle,* and *Confessions of a Kamikaze Cowboy,* by television actor Dirk Benedict.

Unfortunately, too many people who had begun to eat the macrobiotic diet were unable to stay with it. Many people studied hard and prepared healthful meals yet could not successfully make the transition to the diet that they knew could help them. Changing from a diet high in animal foods to a diet high in complex-carbohydrates can create numerous side effects including indigestion, discomfort, gas, and heaviness. The side effects may have resulted from eating the food improperly or may have been part of the body's natural cleansing processes. Overcoming these obstacles is one of the greatest challenges in healing. Too many people gave up the effort.

I know that change is often difficult, even painful. As one adopts a healthier diet, the body will clean out the toxic waste. Uncomfortable symptoms often result. When your cells really begin to cleanse you need to muster all the discipline, knowledge, and positive attitude you can to see you through. To ensure that your transformation will be as smooth as possible, I recommend that you follow the principles of PEP.

My major theory, and the one I am addressing in this book, is that most people who give up the grain-based diet are not eating the food in the manner it must be eaten in order for it to be properly absorbed. *How well you assimilate your food is as important as what you eat.* My success with macrobiotics has been phenomenal. I attribute that largely to my practice of conscious and careful eating, which I first learned from my father.

When I practice the principles of macrobiotics along with the Power Eating Program, I experience profound benefits. Specifically, I develop more energy, calmness, strength, and confidence in myself. More importantly, my enthusiasm for macrobiotics and my satisfaction with whole grains and simple foods continues to increase. I have healed imbalances within myself that, according to Dr. Melvin Page, famed research endocrinologist, would have caused my death long ago. Now I eat to maintain my health, to fulfill my dream, and to be happy. Macrobiotics is a joy and teaching it is a profound honor.

Macrobiotics is neither merely a way of curing illness nor a mystical Oriental cuisine. Some people think it's a brown rice diet, others that it means giving up pleasure at meals. How far from the truth all these ideas are! Macrobiotics is a profound understanding of the orderliness of nature, a practical application which enables us to prepare attractive, delicious meals and achieve a happy and free life.

George Ohsawa
Macrobiotics: An Invitation to Health and Happiness

WHAT IS MACROBIOTICS?

The *Oxford English Dictionary* defines *macrobiotics* as, "Inclined or tending to prolong life; ... The science of prolonging life." Translated from the Greek, macrobiotics means *great life*, or living life to the fullest with joy and health. As an international natural health movement, macrobiotics is:

A PHILOSOPHY of living according to the natural laws of the universe, which are healthy, ecological, and economical.

A PRINCIPLE of understanding energy and how to balance it within ourselves, our foods, our relationships, and in all areas of our lives. This principle is called yin and yang.

A DIET of delicious and satisfying whole organic foods that are nutritionally sound and balanced.

Developed in Japan, modern macrobiotics was founded on ancient health philosophies from the Orient and Europe. Macrobiotic philosophy was carried throughout the world by George Ohsawa and his students Aveline and Michio Kushi, Cornelia and Herman Aihara, Noboru Muramoto, Shizuko Yamamoto and many other teachers. Today, over 500 macrobiotic centers are located internationally.

The purpose of macrobiotics is to help create a more healthy, happy, and peaceful world through the development of personal well-being. Macrobiotics acknowledges many health therapies, including medicine, yet teaches that diet has the most profound power of creating health or illness.

Macrobiotics teaches you how to understand your own unique condition and how to choose foods and lifestyles that can bring you to your optimum state of total health. Taking responsibility for our own life and health is a basic teaching in macrobiotics. Macrobiotic leaders have been pioneers in the natural foods movement throughout the world. Top scientific research institutions have conducted studies regarding the macrobiotic diet and its effect on health.

Countless people worldwide have credited macrobiotics with helping them balance physical and emotional problems. In addition, many others have achieved a deeper spiritual awareness and personal joy through their practice of the macrobiotic way of life.

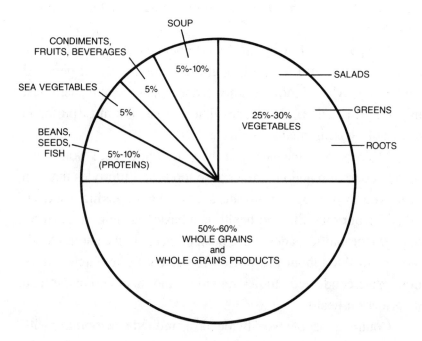

THE STANDARD MACROBIOTIC DIET

The Standard Macrobiotic Diet chart is helpful for instruction yet it is vital to understand that there is not *one* macrobiotic diet. There are many variations, depending on one's needs, conditions, age, climate, profession, and personal goals. Your dietary needs will change as you change. Therefore, it is *essential* to study macrobiotic theory in order to understand your condition and achieve balance. The following list presents the basic categories of healthful foods included in the macrobiotic diet.

WHOLE GRAINS: The foundation of each meal should be 50% to 60% whole grains. Among the delicious, health-giving whole grains are brown rice, whole wheat berries, millet, barley, rye, oats, corn, buckwheat (kasha), quinoa, and amaranth. Whole-grain products such as bulghur, oatmeal, noodles, corn grits, sourdough whole wheat bread, chapaties, and sprouted grain bread are also included.

SOUP: Standard macrobiotic guidelines suggest one or two small bowls of vegetable soup, comprising approximately 5% to 10% of your daily food intake. The soup is prepared with land and sea vegetables along with savory miso or tamari added as a delicious, mild seasoning and as a tremendous nutrition boost.

VEGETABLES: Fresh, organic vegetables, prepared in a variety of ways compose 25% to 30% of a standard diet. From steamed vegetables to stir-fried vegetables, from crispy salads to rich stews, vegetables are versatile and vital for our health.

BEANS: An excellent protein, mineral, and fiber source, beans and bean products are recommended as 5% to 10% of our daily food. Prepared with sea vegetables and grains, or in soups and salads, beans are hearty, satisfying and delicious.

SEA VEGETABLES: These vitamin- and mineral-rich foods supply important nutrients lacking in the American farmlands and foods. Comprising about 5% of our diet, sea vegetables are eaten daily in beans, soups, vegetables, and even desserts.

SUPPLEMENTAL FOODS

SEEDS AND NUTS: Roasted sesame, pumpkin, and sunflower seeds are an integral part of the macrobiotic diet that supply valuable minerals and high-quality protein. Nuts and nut butters are to be used sparingly.

FISH: Occasionally, a moderate amount (3-5 ounces) of white-meat fish and seafood is desirable for some people once or twice a week or as needed. When eating fish, I recommend consuming three times more vegetables than fish, and including a small raw salad and high-quality dessert.

DESSERTS AND SWEETENERS: Grain-based sweeteners such as rice syrup, barley malt, and amasake are preferred. A variety of pies, cakes, cookies, puddings, and gelatins are prepared with these sweeteners and eaten in moderation. Fruit juices may be used as sweeteners on occasion.

FRUITS: Depending on one's condition, needs, and climate, local fruits in season are recommended in moderate amounts.

COOKING OIL: Naturally processed, cold-pressed vegetable oils are recommended in cooking a great variety of tasty dishes. Solid or saturated fats and margarines are avoided.

CONDIMENTS: The array of healthful condiments are vital additions to the macrobiotic diet that help people adjust the taste and medicinal quality of their foods. I highly recommend the careful study and use of valuable condiments such as gomashio (sesame salt), umeboshi plums, tekka, and sea vegetable powders. Sea salt is best used sparingly in cooking and with knowledge of its effects.

PICKLES: Fermented vegetable pickles eaten daily are natural digestive aids which help to alkalize the body and to provide healthy intestinal functions.

BEVERAGES: Spring or well water is recommended for drinking, and in the preparation of food and teas. Often, filtered water is preferred for its economy and convenience. Bancha tea, roasted grain teas, and non-stimulant herbal teas are the most frequently served beverages. Avoid iced beverages.

The Standard Macrobiotic Diet contains a tremendous variety of foods and cooking styles. Please read some of the marvelous, comprehensive macrobiotic cookbooks currently available that list specific foods, detail their values, and provide abundant recipes for delicious, powerful and healthful meals. Take macrobiotic cooking classes and learn to prepare the foods you and your family need for optimum wellness. For a healthy, happy balance, macrobiotic study is essential.

(The original Standard Macrobiotic Diet and Way of Life Suggestions were developed and published by the Kushi Institute, Brookline, Massachusetts.)

MACROBIOTIC WAY-OF-LIFE SUGGESTIONS

- Cultivate a positive attitude as you live a happy and active life.
- Spend at least one hour outdoors each day but avoid the strong noon sun.
- Learn to prepare delicious natural foods that balance you and your family.
- Create peaceful mealtimes.
- Chew your food well.
- Take a walk outside daily, preferably barefoot on the grass, beach, or earth.
- Several times a week, exercise to the point of sweating as you dance, bicycle, walk, or do an enjoyable activity.
- Try to go to bed by 11:00 p.m. and rise at sunrise.
- Put order into your house by cleaning and organizing each area.
- Make sure your clothing and bed linens are made of natural fibers.
- Avoid chemicals and other environmental pollutants in your home and workplace. Use healthy alternatives when possible.
- Bring natural, green plants into your home and office to oxygenate and freshen the air.
- Open your house daily to let fresh air inside.
- Stimulate your entire body daily with a hot-towel self-massage.
- A flame or gas stove is essential. Avoid electric or microwave cooking.
- Use a protective screen on your color television and computer terminal.
- Communicate frequently with others, sharing feelings and learning about yourself and your world.
- Appreciate yourself, discover and utilize your talents and find a life-work that brings you joy.
- Develop a sense of gratitude about the precious life we are given.

TOGETHER ON THE JOURNEY...

I am continuing to experiment and discover many things about eating and chewing. Something magical happens when I practice PEP. Many people have told me how their lives have improved since they began eating in a conscious manner. I would be happy to hear about your experiences with the Power Eating Progam. I encourage you to eat the best diet, balanced for your unique needs, and to practice PEP. Then share your results and benefits with your friends.

The greatest, most healing changes in this world will be made by you and me, as we perform the most simple, yet profound actions of our daily life. The main ingredients for miracles are right under our noses–three times a day. Our food and the way we eat it is powerfully affecting our lives and the survival of this beautiful planet.

I lovingly pass along to you the advice my father gave me one day when I was young, on a picnic in Yugoslavia. "If ever you are weak, cold, or sick, chew each mouthful 150 times or more." This advice could help save thousands of lives among the millions of people throughout the world who are starving and suffering illness at this very moment.

May we grow together in consciousness and save our Mother Earth before it is too late. May we love ourselves enough to give our minds and bodies the healthiest foods, both physical and spiritual. May you, my friend, realize your life dream as you enjoy a life of health, happiness, and peace in the realization of your fullest power.

HAPPY CHEWING!

Lino

PEP SONG

CHEW, CHEW, CHEW YOUR FOOD
GENTLY THROUGH THE MEAL
THE MORE YOU CHEW THE LESS YOU EAT
THE BETTER YOU WILL FEEL!

(To be sung to the tune of "Row, Row, Row Your Boat")

BIBLIOGRAPHY

Aihara, Herman. *Basic Macrobiotics*. Tokyo and New York: Japan Publications, Inc.,1985.

_____."Essence of Body Health: The Liver and Kidneys." *Macrobiotics Today*. Oroville, California: George Ohsawa Macrobiotic Foundation, June, 1989.

Brody, Jane. *Jane Brody's Nutrition Book*. New York, New York: Bantam Books, 1982.

"Consumer Spending Report." *Drug Topics*: Oradelle, N.J., July 1, 1985.

Diet, Nutrition, and Cancer. National Academy of Sciences. Washington, D.C.: 1982.

Dietary Goals for the United States. Select Committee on Nutrition and Human Needs. Washington, D.C.: 1977

Fox, Philip C. "Saliva Inhibits HIV-1 Infectivity." *The Journal of the American Dental Association*. Volume 116, No. 6, May 1988, 635.

Ganzfried, Rabbi Solomon. *Code of Jewish Law*. Brooklyn, New York: Hebrew Publishing Company, 1963.

Haas, Robert. *Eat To Win, The Sports Nutrition Bible*. New York, New York: Rawson Associates, 1983.

Kushi, Michio and Alex Jack. *The Book of Macrobiotics*. Tokyo and New York, New York: Japan Publications, Inc., 1986.

Kuntzleman, Charles T., and Editors of Consumer Guide. *The Complete Book of Walking*. New York, New York: Simon & Schuster, Inc., 1982.

Loehr, James E. and Jeffrey A. Migdow. *Take A Deep Breath.* New York, New York: Villard Books, 1986.

Muktananda, Swami. *Reflections of the Self,* Part I, v. 198. South Fallsburg, New York: SYDA Foundation, 1980.

_____.*Satsang With Baba,* Vol. I. South Fallsburg, New York: SYDA Foundation, 1974.

Muramoto, Noboru. *Natural Immunity : Insights on Diet and AIDS.* Oroville, California: George Ohsawa Macrobiotic Foundation, 1988.

Ohsawa, George. *An Invitation to Health and Happiness.* Oroville, California: George Ohsawa Macrobiotic Foundation, 1971.

_____.*Practical Guide to Far Eastern Macrobiotic Medicine.* Oroville, California: George Ohsawa Macrobiotic Foundation, 1976.

Quincannon, Jane. "Roots To Infinity." *Return To Paradise.* Beckett, Massachusetts: Kushi Foundation for One Peaceful World, Spring 1989, 8-9.

Robbins, Anthony. *Unlimited Power.* New York, New York: Ballantine Books, 1986.

Robbins, John. *Diet For A New America.* Walpole, New Hampshire: Stillpoint Publishing, 1987.

Rossoff, Michael. "Finding Piece of Mind in Troubled Times." *Solstice.* Charlottesville, Virginia: Volume 36, May/June (1989), 12-14.

Siegel, Bernie S. *Love, Medicine and Miracles*. New York, New York: Harper & Row, Publishers, 1986.

Szekely, Edmond Bordeaux. *The Essene Gospel of Peace*. Cartago, Costa Rica: I.B.S. International, 1981.

Tara, William. "Making Macrobiotics Work For You." *The Joy of Life*. Coconut Grove, Florida: The Macrobiotic Foundation of Florida: Spring 1989, 35.

Taylor, Renee. *Hunza Health Secrets*. New York, New York: Award Books, 1964.

"We're Eating Our Way To Early Graves, U.S. Says." *Miami News*, July 27, 1988.

Yamamoto, Shizuko. *Barefoot Shiatsu*. New York, New York: Japan Publications, 1979.

Yogananda, Paramahansa. *Scientific Healing Affirmations*. Los Angeles, California: Self-Realization Fellowship, 1981.

ABOUT THE AUTHOR

Lino Stanchich is a Kushi Institute Certified Senior Macrobiotic Counselor and Teacher. He has studied and worked with the world's foremost wholistic health practitioners and educators. For the past twenty years, Mr. Stanchich has taught Macrobiotics, Oriental Diagnosis and Medicine, Nutrition, Massage, Exercise and Special Eating Techniques to students, physicians and health professionals, as well as to individuals and families. Mr. Stanchich has appeared on television and radio programs promoting natural health. He regularly teaches at macrobiotic centers and conferences in the United States and Europe.

Founder of Walden Center in Providence, Rhode Island, and of the Tucson East West Center/Ranch in Tucson, Arizona, Lino Stanchich was also Director of Asunaro Institute in Escondido, California. He was co-founder of two natural foods businesses; Herb T Company and Great Life Products. Mr. Stanchich is also a health consultant to executives in professional organizations and corporations. He conducts macrobiotic and Power Eating Program seminars for a worldwide audience.

NOTES

ORDER FORM

EVERYONE EATS! Since everyone wants more health and energy, *Power Eating Program* makes a wonderful gift for friends and family. Here is a form for easy ordering. Please print clearly.

RATES

Quantity Ordered	P.E.P. (per copy)	Shipping & Handling (per copy)		RUSH Shipping (per copy)
One copy	$9.95	+ $2.00	OR	$3.00
10 or more copies	$6.95	+ $1.00	OR	$1.50

Quantity Ordered			Amount Enclosed
	Copy(s) Power Eating Program @ $9.95 each	=	$.
	10 or more copies @ $6.95 each	=	.
	Shipping and Handling @ $_____ per copy	=	.
	Florida residents only, please add 6% sales tax		.
	· TOTAL ENCLOSED		$.

Your Name and Address | Shipping Name and Address (if different from your own)

Name	
Address	
City, ST, Zip	
Telephone	

Please indicate method of payment:

☐ CHECK   ☐ MONEY ORDER

Make check or money order payable to:

HEALTHY PRODUCTS, INC.

Send To: P.O. Box 19315
Asheville, North Carolina 28815
(828) 299-8657

PEP is a book you can really sink your teeth into!

HEALTHY PRODUCTS ORDER FORM

New and exciting educational materials by Lino Stanchich are now available.

NEW!   MACROBIOTIC HEALING SECRETS, VOL. I

Lino's newest book provides essential information about crucial topics that will make a difference in the success of your macrobiotic practice, your health and your life: SLEEP, NIGHTSHADES, CANDIDA, DISCHARGING, CRAVINGS, SUPER ENERGY, FERMENTED FOODS.

QUANTITY	PRICE	SHIPPING & HANDLING PER COPY
1 Book	$ 13.95	$4.00 (U.S.A.), $6.00 (Canada)
10+ Books	$ 8.50	$1.00 (U.S.A.), $3.00 (Canada)

HEALING MEALTIME MUSIC CASSETTE and CD

Soothing piano melodies with a bell, as a gentle reminder to chew your food well. Beautiful, original music, composed by Will Tuttle, Ph.D., under the direction of Lino Stanchich, creates a peaceful mealtime atmosphere, proven to promote better digestion, and improved health. Useful in conjunction with the *Power Eating Program*. 90 minutes.

QUANTITY	PRICE	SHIPPING & HANDLING PER COPY
1 cassette	$ 9.95	$4.00 (U.S.A.), $6.00 (Canada)
1 CD	$14.95	(Same as above.)

ENERGIZE YOURSELF WITH SELF-MASSAGE! VIDEO

Have a lifetime of daily massages given by your best friend-YOURSELF! Wake up your vitality the fun, easy way! Filmed outdoors on a beautiful Colorado mountain-side, Lino Stanchich expertly teaches, step by step, a total body self-massage (Do In). 55 minutes.

QUANTITY	PRICE	SHIPPING & HANDLING PER COPY
1 Video	$ 25.00	$4.00 (U.S.A.), $6.00 (Canada)
2-10 Videos	$ 22.00	$3.00 (U.S.A.), $4.00 (Canada)

LAUGH! For the Health of It, Audio

Laughter truly is one of the best medicines. If you are unhappy, unhealthy, or want more joy in life, this audio is for you! Jane and Lino are tickled to give you and your family the tools to laugh more each day. Laugh along with Lino. Laughter has been proven to:

- Decrease Pain
- Reduce Stress
- Improve Circulation
- Decrease Anger
- Lower Blood Pressure
- Strengthen Immunity
- Dispel Depression
- Increase Joy of Life

QUANTITY	PRICE	SHIPPING & HANDLING
1 cassette	$ 10.95	$ 4.00 (USA), $6.00 (Canada)
1 CD	$ 14.95	(Same as above)

Send check or money order to:
HEALTHY PRODUCTS, INC., 101 Willow Lake Drive, Asheville, NC 28805
Phone (828) 299-8657   Fax (828) 299-8658

Visit our web site: macrobioticconsultation.com